ARTS OF PALEO-FASTING

Magic Door of the Superior Man

Karen Kellock Ph.D.

This book series is dedicated to
children and animals: the innocent will of God
and to all God's elect making amazing new dents.
For breakthrough, just fast (fly), separate and repent!

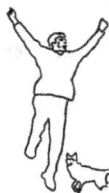

I lost my health for decades but now
I have it in spades cuz I overcame the
Ideological shovedown since the sixties.
Carnivores eat fruit and leaves:
It's a matter of *proportion*, which varies.

FORMULA:

All success attraction
All disease obstruction
All recovery elimination

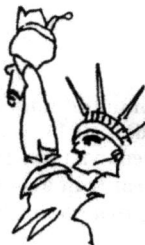

You must fast on all three

OBSTRUCTIONS:

People
Habit
Food

ARTS OF PALEO-FASTING

Magic Door of the Superior Man

PREFACE: OBSTRUCTION

1   Transformation

2   Sacred Fat-Fast

3   Happy Fat-Fast

4   Feast or Fast

5   Ectos-Free

6   Depression

7   Bore-Dumb

8   Ana Sage

9   Glamorous Aging

10   Worry

11   Loneliness

Paleo Power and Obligate Carnivores

Selfhood Obstructions

Lascivious Liberalism

Frightening Feminists

Hostile Invasion of Young Men

APPENDICES

Must fast on all obstructions:
People, Habit and Food

Key-locks

Big Ten

Speak KK

Art and Science Discovery

High-Fat is High-Tech

Questions on Fatarianism

Study of A Cerebrotonic Introvert Overcomer

Bibliography

Author Bio

PREFACE: OBSTRUCTION

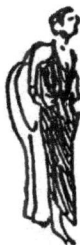

In the Act of Creation Koestler showed how landmark discoveries link with history—as part of nature, would this not be true? We all have a unique talent, the seed of a creative act inside--but it's a mere potential. It must be developed to blossom into world-changing power. Completion is natural and synchronicity is intelligent design but this natural process in man is *blocked by obstruction:* people, habits and food. If pure, the creative act evolves through cycles: it sprouts, moves into place and completes itself naturally. Timing is all: the minute the act is complete the link appears. Just by fasting and doing what comes naturally our true genius comes through: we do magical work for magical pay. The test of discovery is: does it work?

Human functioning has most to do with *released obstruction* from non-essentials but you also need animal fat: "fauna". If you've a world destiny and you can't get that final breakthrough after years of thankless effort, then fauna-fasting is the last brick of that building--the one thing you haven't done. If you say "but I've fasted lunch" then you must do more to get that final hunch--tighten your belt further. This could mean bailing from a sick relationship or an old (outdated, useless) habit that must now go. For the time is late--it's with destiny you have a date. It's time you are ready to show for dough (by looking like a doe--it means living like Thoreau). If you want your success to be more than a comet— an overnight success then a splash (no finesse or an excess-mess)--then let DAILY FASTING (on food, people and bad habits) along with solitude establish your new foundation. You must now be a cute decoration to achieve your final coronation.

The Struggles of Genius in Overcoming Obstruction.
Your Time Will Come If You Faint Not.

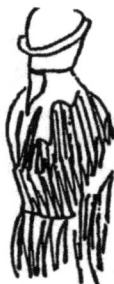

Take fruit or fat then fast twenty hours, releasing all powers. Or eat mouse meals—continuous fasting punctuated by bites. Thus return to selfhood and success, your rights. If fasting, Human Growth Hormone is released at night. It youthifies, repairs and fills you with might. People and habits: Clean sweep precedes success. Cut it all loose, then God will bless. Champs have a destiny and clarity puts them on the crest. Just fast on all obstruction then do your best.

The DAILY FAST is always rewarded

You'll see your digestion, assimilation, elimination (and thus appearance) improve as all hunger dissolves. All your problems you'll find this solves. You will have a slim and strong body, vivid lucid perception, keen discernment, energy to work all day (starting before dawn) and total success. Each dawn is a new beginning so forget the past and try again, soon you'll get it right.

PALEOFASTER'S FIX (RX):

The paleo foods are fruits, vegetables, meat, nuts and berries. The high-fat diet is high-tech for it's so easy to fast after fauna: animal protein and fat. You will be amazed how satiated you'll feel for one or two days. You'll feel so good daily fasting will become your new addiction. From that will spring an interest in all other things and life will catapult up. To remove this stumbling block through the daily fast is to explode their life into new and higher dimensions.

Fat-Fast

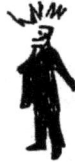

Welcome to the highest life possible:

PALEO-FASTING

Paleo-fasting is a magic door you step into by the mere decision to fast. The superior man knows that whatever the problem, just by fasting he enters this door where his foes fall to the floor, he changes to the core and to the fast he says "I want more!"   Now you enter cornucopia and the stars look so bright in a fast: Just by skipping dinner the senses explode open to vast   perception. Not-digesting we gain high fidelity to an abundant environment and the nights are as exciting as the days. This miraculous new adventure is revealed to the daily fastarian free of people, habit and food obstructions. To decrease (fast on all three) is to increase (magnify experience)—the more micro our attention the more macro our experience. This is:

FastGlorious

TRANSFORMATION
Chaos Benefits the Party Not in Power
So Remove Obstructions for the Time is Dire

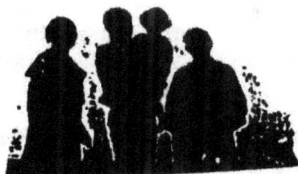

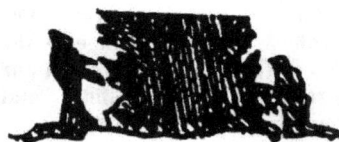

After so much obstruction, resistance and people working against you finally we arrive at clarity, or glamorous aging. This is growing into your own skin—becoming more *yourself* as the years pass. This is magnetic, charismatic and perfect. It's like finding a brand new life as a five year old, totally spontaneous and creative. As you clear up from false roles each moment is blissful, flamboyant and lucid with new sights and sounds. The glamorous elder's days are packed-in with ecstatic enjoyment: intense happiness from overcoming pain and distress. To partake of this bliss remove the obstructions and get ready for transformation--a striking alteration in appearance and character. Though so many years have passed you'll be younger than before the fast.

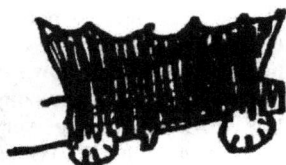

High-tech society has not changed human nature—it's the same as the horse and buggy days for living in society is now a *gag rule*: restricted freedom of debate or expression. But once free our lives take on *gaiety*: merrymaking of spirits like a child. Then we *gain*: win in competition of conflict. Free of obstruction, we *get* by a natural development or process: we achieve and attract attention, profit, increase and health. We become a "heavy" and *gainful*: graceful, magnetic, attractive and *galactic* (relating to the galaxy). It's a matter of God's design—we become *galatea*, like an ivory statue

ARTS OF PALEO FASTING

of a maiden carved by Pygmalion. It takes time but this is becoming paleo, or *galax*: like evergreen decorative leaves. This is elder beauty, personal firepower or glamour as we become part of the galaxy: assemblage of brilliant or notable persons. This is the opposite to the old life of *gale*: emotional outbursts, galimatias: confused and meaningless talk or gibberish and *gall*-- bitter things to endure or rancor of spirit. The old life started to gall: fret, irritate, vex, harass and wear away our joy but this provided the necessary friction and heat to make *gold*: refine our spirits from grossness to purity. With glamorous aging we wear a symbolic *galea*: the helmet of victory--we have "panache".

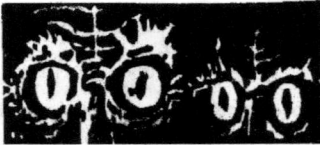

The opposite of transformation is staying stuck in the muck, and as we age these templates harden into fear. But the result of transformation is being *meta*: a later or more highly organized specialized form. For this metamorphosis is like a change in the constitution of rock affected by pressure—we've used the catastrophe in our life to force a change to a more highly crystalline and compact condition. This physical newness occurs by supernatural means and it's bound to shock our associates, for through the fast (on food, people and habits) we've changed our chemistry, texture, tissues, every cell and our circumstances--drastically and suddenly.

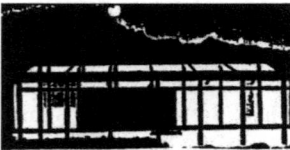

The results are like the marked or abrupt change subsequent to birth or hatching: suddenly a whole new matrix appears. It makes one metaphysical—transcendent or supernatural--so that our lives become poetic: marked by elaborate subtleties of thought and expression. This is becoming rich! We rebuild the house by cutting down to the core then adding on the new elements galore. To bring on this amazing transfiguration we use a method: the DAILY FAST--choosing very carefully what gets in body, mind, spirit and home. Our diet and lifestyle is FF: Fauna-Fastarianism.

SLOW BUT STEADY
Invisibly You're Getting Ready

ARTS OF PALEO FASTING

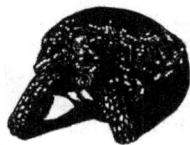

Growth may seem slow but it's steady, for underground (invisibly) we're getting ready. Because of the radically stepped-up alteration in your humdrum life you will become delightfully addicted to fasting and eventually become mestiza—like a different culture: brown, thin, lustrous (with iridescent plumage. the sign of a true leader) and mestoa—a later and more complex form of life which is blissful and silent. As the sticky starchy sludge dislodges from the cell wall the skin becomes tightly woven as the new blood shows through--a darker complexion manifests. By sticking to this strict but enjoyable method your tastes change and each day you have cleaner tissues, less hunger, more beauty and fascination with life as you graduate into this higher grade of neanthropic hyper-evolution, the look and feel of high-tech futurism. At this point you'll become like a farmer--instinctively knowing the coming seasons. Since everything is a matter of timing you'll know when to plant, when to harvest-- when to speak and when to be silent. That's how you'll win: hands down (no more spin). This connectedness is utter bliss and happiness from (unblocked) clear energy--not frozen or recycled energy (sin). Now just go with the flow and don't force your own puny petty plans--you're part of something higher now. Just fast and accept all delays as the fastest route. Then learn to see through images--for whether churchmen or alcoholic they all must repent for success to occur (or stay in a blur). Lastly, know the value of leisure--that's when revelations occur, for sure.

LEAVE A SPACE : PNEUMATICITY
Attracting Stronger Elements

Fasting is a celestial law making you celestial grade with celestial attractions of strong elements for a change. You don't have to have strength to create your flamboyant destiny—all you have to do is *fast and let that bring it all in.* You'll progress by whirling into new dimensions as you release obstruction, for clearing away space acts as a magnet filling it in with new higher things: this is the principal of *pneumaticity*. For this solid, bullish strength in foundation you don't have to do anything else but fast--for now you'll rule by attraction, not fighting in factions. Close old doors, new ones open so just "leave a space". When fasting close one and five open as everything accelerates. This exciting trip is exteroceptive—a sensory journey from which there is no return, like sitting in an astrodome for celestial observations. By your mere decision to fast you have changed the influence of the stars upon your human affairs, as

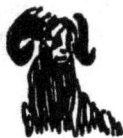

your new astrophysical gravitation is a choice: Make a space then attract all due to the law of affinitization (like-attracting-like in the pulls of gravity). Now you can have the perfect *pulling* power of the most talented people in the race. God has given us this method to change the stars so anything can be changed, nothing is hopeless, and nothing is etched in stone. Whether in pit or prison, you'll soon be in a palace—as your star is shown you'll become well-known as destiny arrives full-blown.

HEALING THE SPLIT
Opening to Spirit: Throwbacks

It hurts to be split, as power and beauty fades and we lose identity--or become a dark knight lost in the primitive (collective) subconscious. Man has two sides and the more energy he has at birth the more he goes way up (renowned) or just as far down (the clown). This energy is either self-expressive or self-destructive--making gold heals this split so the shattered forces (and the resulting flagged fascination with life) unite into a rod of power, creativity and perfect success. The best saints were the worst sinners and so with repentance their lives showed sudden emergence on the world scene after decades of dung and dryness. To be a success we must focus and eliminate all distraction--and through the fast we have. The mental changes are as sudden as the physical as we become astute: sagacious, wily, shrewd. This brings on an atavism—a trait more typical of ancestors but remote from parents and siblings due to a recombination of ancestral genes—we become a throwback. Suddenly we can't relate to those still hooked to culture as we mentally transport to new worlds in pure rapture. We transformed because we were *fusible*: like an alloy having a melting point our fusion resulted from the heat produced by life's pressures and irritations combined with the refusal to give into the food-fix. This is the refinement process of making gold: eliminating our gross aspects (ignobility) and becoming refined (true nobility). The fragments of your personality have now merged into one--the glamorous elder--and this fusion of atomic energy brings a world fuss: effusive praise.

PHANTASMAGORIA
High Boundaries Brings Rapture

ARTS OF PALEO FASTING

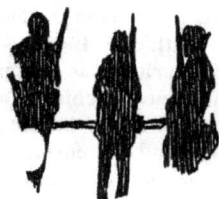

Now strong we're no longer a victim of the forces of fate or hostile environments. Now impervious to the nervous and the imperious, we create not just *react* and so our vision explodes to a fantasiacal perception. Living within high boundaries (insulated within a hedge of protection) life becomes a phantasmagoria as we move from one frame to the next, appreciating everything in sequence. Opening up to nature, the universe, the moment and God will thrill your soul, whereas you were left-brained in reactive stress (it took its toll). Getting away from the petty details of everyday life will make you so happy every day and through the daily fast you'll stay that way. You must eliminate obstructions and distractions and then keep them away. Now just establish your own best routine according to the seasons of the day--move from one pool to the next, letting fullness of life be your text. Learn to appreciate leisure: that's living the seasonal way, for even work becomes play if it's in the proper time of day--your peak period when everything pays.

CAN'T PULL 'EM UP TOO
Find a New Stew

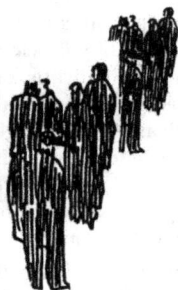

While you've become glamorously ageless your peers are still *fusty* with age: impaired, damp, moldy, saturated with dust and stale orders (musty)--old-fashioned or rigidly conservative. They've become *futile*: serving no useful purpose, occupied with trifles and frivolous. Unlike you they have no *future*: expectation of advancement or progressive development. You are future perfect and they are not, being immersed in *fuzz*: enveloped in a haze, a blur, looseness, laxness, spongy, rotten and foul—unclear, indistinct. But you've been salvaged from the mass for like all saints and sages in history the fast moved you closer to God—more Godlike. You've become beautiful through revelation-evacuation: As the clogged colon spills sludge the entire system clarifies (de-ages) and you see everything differently—all problems are solved (if your cycles and systems stay resolved).

FAST INTO PERFECTION: KEYSTONE

ARTS OF PALEO FASTING

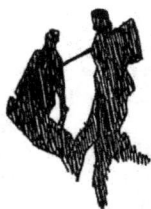

As you become more receptive to God you become more perfect--released from culture yet protected then elected. This is becoming like the mythical Indian—mysterious, strong, silent--yet more worldly as deep archetypes are released (exemplar, sultan, pharaoh, chief). In opening up to timeless space and time you become magnificent: in dignity (good taste) and imposing—impressive. You become stately in your poised dignity, erectness of bearing, handsomeness of proportions, and ceremoniously majestic comportment of grandeur. You are now a colorful cornucopia of God's beautiful nature, love, joy and the magic of the creative spirit. You've become the keystone: the uppermost stone of an arch completing and locking all its members together, and this is your crowning achievement.

GENETIC BODY FLUIDS

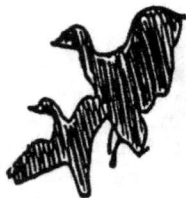

Now you're part of God's nature—instinctively perfect—not degraded through human nature: bad reflect, the least you could expect, with disrespect (a sad reject). The daily fast makes you exquisite: a diamond cut of perfection after so much deformation. This is being majestic or illustrious: the exquisite spirit is choice, accurate, marked by flawless craftsmanship or by beautiful, ingenious, delicate or elaborate execution. You've become keenly appreciative, discriminating and accomplished--pleasing through beauty, fitness or perfection, acuteness and intensity. A "diamond cut" is called "brilliant" due to numerous facets cut for special brilliancy. And so we always look forward to our fasting selfix: Knowing the body snaps back into perfection brings so much joy and assurance. Key: fast. Pop: lock into new dimensions composed of all of your multi-talents. You take on *genetic body fluids*: the best traits of all of your ancestors manifested in you--the finest final stew. (This comes after eradicating all the worst traits accumulated in you.) This perfect constellation of the diamond comes from pressure from all sides which finally puts you into perfect shape. Whew--after being so blue through the daily fast we're brand new (only this is true).

RESILIENCY SHOOTS TO INFINITY
Not Stuck in "Bad Luck"

ARTS OF PALEO FASTING

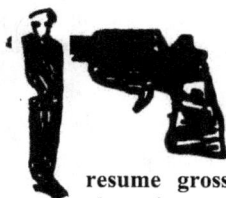

Having made gold we are the power of a gun in the body politic. As champions we have an *elastic* nature: capable of recovering size and shape after deformation, capable of indefinite expansion and recovering quickly from depression or disappointment, capable of being easily stretched and expanded and careful not to resume grosser shapes (having learned from our mistakes). We champions are the resilient: recovering quickly when deforming pressure (food, people, habit) is removed. We *spring*: after yielding to the pressure we quickly return to our original shape. We are *supple*: bent, twisted or folded without sign or injury. We are elves and Indian angels: thin, fragile, glossy, efflorescing chemically with redness of skin and poised yet with unheard-of courage, boldness and energy in public life. We are now suited up for the crown, ever-ready for creative action. This effervescence is liveliness and exhilaration, and what a trip as we've become illustrious: obviously famous, notably or brilliantly outstanding and eminent: shining brightly with light--clear evidence of fame, renown or notoriety.

BECOMING A RED INDIAN

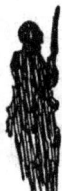

There are different states of energy vs. radioactive decay. These radioactive transformations exhibit velocity of light transmission and this is the fasting process. So hold on--each day you'll be more energy efficient and unique (different from the mass). Now you're a happy gentleman or lass, an Indian protected with high boundaries: red, humming, buzzing and effervescing chemically by a clean bloodstream and thoughts as clear as the sky with no distractions. Indians are always happy, ecstatically ever-mindful of the changes in nature--and fasting is our path to these galactic revelations and viewpoints, handsome proportions, stately posture, elegant grace and fine features (a symmetrical crystal). When the obstruction is removed you see everything differently-- you've gone from spiritual darkness to God's light, a fine crystal made perfect from living right.

When "up" in the crown charka your hair resembles the laureate leaf—lustrous and majestic marking the true leader. But when down you may look dumb. Now fast and let the posture elongate while your vision expands into nature and the future. The further from the last meal the less hunger, and the more you'll have separated from your peers. For a Godlike life is glamorous agelessness: loving, clean, sacred, pure, colorful, bountiful, magnetic and beautiful: this is "high". The opposite way is how the herd ages into ugliness, stodginess, fear and addictions—blocked energy making one dense, drugged, down or disgraced.

HOW TO MAKE GOLD: FAST AND WAIT
More beautiful with Age—You're Becoming the Sage

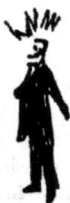

Anyone can be a success. The problem is not how to get to success but how to handle it when we get there. Cosmic man does nothing— he *attracts* what he is. Because he has peace he has total power. By doing nothing but fasting (on people, habit and food) he clears up the system by de-cluttering it from meaningless details dimming his light. From clutter to clarity, he snaps to his goal. Through the daily fast he goes from an ordinary man to an extraordinary genius living in timelessness. Cosmic man watches for miracles like a cat watches a mouse-hole: he just sits quietly while the ever-changing puzzle comes together. This is the reality of children, saints and geniuses in a magic cornucopia: a colorful land of miracles dancing on the cycles of nature. The creative act is like a jigsaw puzzle falling together in a pattern: the perfect plan of a unique destiny. Einstein had this sense of "cosmic religiousness": awe and wonder at a perfectly-ordered universe where everything fits (if we don't force the fit). Cosmic man has learned this from obstacles overcome (being misunderstood and rejected) for he is the cornerstone, the "stone the builder's rejected"—overlooked as useless, worthless and of no value. Overcoming this obstacle unleashes surplus potentials: Genius is born of problematic soil but flourishes only in nonproblematic soil. These are the simple keys so now just take your victory if you please then thank God on your knees.

UNIQUE SEED SYMBOL

At birth our unique seed symbol contains all of our potentials--this is the opposing force at any moment to be seen in clarity as everything that is ours by divine right snaps in. Fasting reverts to type as the configuration of our energies converge in this perfect pattern. The seed symbol is the true self: eternal, boundless and ageless and all else is deformation of this perfection. The seed is our divine election bringing God's and man's affection.

ARCHETYPES ARE THE KEYS

ARTS OF PALEO FASTING

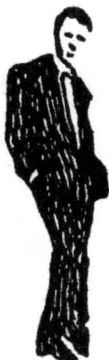

It is the archetypes, or symbols of self which are the keys unlocking these powers of attraction. Any behavior which degrades the symbol brings inferior attractions. We attract what we *are*, not what we say we are. Archetypes are the keys unlocking heaven and locking down hell as everything falls together in good vs. bad patterns dependent on our clarity vs. denseness. The champion has learned what keeps him clear and how not to go dense again. The key: fast and purify for success in all pursuits. With the mere decision PHF (positive healing forces) are released, the deformation passes, our seed symbol emerges and we're locked in a higher dimension (with no return of old jealousies or hates). In this high gear it's over all problems and disruptions he skates for now he hums (not grates): as a Co-creator with God not a victim of mean fates.

☐☐PETTY STANDARDS TO COMPETE

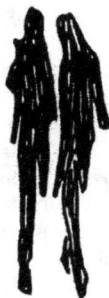

When our energies deform we fall in with social hypnotism and take on herd (cultural) stereotypes and petty standards to compete rather than the universal archetypes magnetizing our success by attraction alone. In truth there is nothing to do, or no one to see. Just continue to clear up until that moment success occurs--the great divide into pure paradise. Superior man conforms to no one since he's totally unique (one-of-a-kind). He has learned that to conform is to bloat out and bog down--become ordinary. He knows he is made superior by taming his instincts for the biological ones become compulsive. Making Gold is becoming a knight (over self) and this is: extraordinary. Why, he asks, should he compete with the petty when all he has to do is do his genius? So he just does his work and leaves the rest of the day for relaxation and inspiration: this will be his pattern for the rest of his long, luxurious life. For in the twinkling of an eye the old miserable life is gone forever and the new panoramic life of happiness has begun, and thus the goal of all spiritual teachings if to find his true self as pre-designed by God—the unchanging pure philosopher's stone as solid and unique as the rock of Gibraltar. This is the "treasure hard to attain" for usually it takes prolonged years of suffering to burn away the gross elements.

SACRED FAT-FAST

God satisfieth thy mouth with good things so thy youth
is renewed like the eagles. Psalms 103: 5

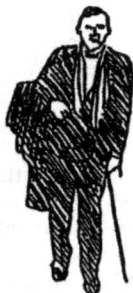

Fasting after protein and fat evokes HGH which returns us to youth. Enjoy
thy week-end fat-fast and stay ageless until the very end. It's so enjoyable
you'll be starting week-ends on Wednesdays.

HUMAN GROWTH HORMONE: YOUTH

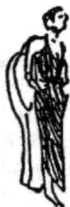

The key to superior health and maximum longevity is HGH: Human
Growth Hormone. This "master hormone" maintains, repairs and
rebuilds every cell and tissue while returning us to youth, no matter
what our age. HGH keeps people "full of life" and free of disease. It
keeps them young: elevating energy and burning fat while reducing
stress and insulin resistance. HGH produces "growth factors" of
youth--and though it declines after twenty and extremely so after
forty it is produced despite advanced age through fasting first, and
animal protein second. And so the sacred weekend fast begins with
protein like a cheese omelet then a pain-free fast after which you'll say "I had
a blast".

ARTS OF PALEO FASTING

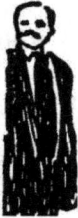

As HGH decreases with age the body enters the catabolic state of breakdown and disrepair: aging. The body's anabolic state (growth, repair, youth) becomes catabolic. Any stimulation of HGH (like fasting) reverses this aging process while wrong eating inhibits HGH and accelerates it. Excessive levels of HGH occur after just a three-day fasting week-end, so that even in very old age the person literally and quickly becomes young again. Food-limitation brings amazing youthification—a de-aging process which is so astounding that even at 70 or 80 one becomes a young child and longevity is doubled! Any age can be revived (see: Gandhi when old). The elderly can secrete as much growth hormone as the young but only fasting releases it after 40. With the sacred fasting weekend old and young alike are renewed and that means beautiful—you're ready to be viewed whereas on Friday you looked crude.

CALORIE-RESTRICTED DIETS AND HGH
Magic Week-End Fat-Fast

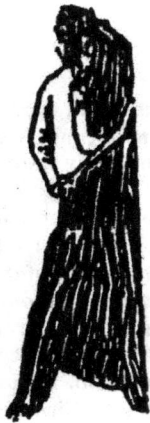

Anabolic: youth and repair. Catabolic: breakdown and dis-repair. Animals on calorie-restricted diets live twice as long and actually get much younger even late in life. After eating small meals of fat one is appetite-suppressed for long periods and he can easily fast--paleo foods and fasting just go together so on week-ends we fast ala Atkins all the way. Whether recovering from a fight or just needing the light you can elevate the anabolic tonight as all wrongs become right. You'll be amazed at how full you feel after a cordon bleu and this satiety will last the whole weekend. Fasting is a "hyper-anabolic" state taking us back to youth with full resilience—it is hormones which determine which state we are in. The vegan community will never admit that animal foods keep us young—they just can't take this info on the chin (they're no fun)—but it's the hormone glucagons (from fauna) which puts on humans a grin. During the fast HGH becomes excessive: just three days shows miraculous elevation while wrong-eating (starch/sugar/fiber/processed) decreases it completely. When fasting we live on ketones: our own inessential flesh (fat and debris) so that even with complete starvation the body saves the brain, spinal cord, lungs, and heart for last and even then it works on them very slowly. Don't worry: fast, get thin, be happy and strong and avoid the throng—they are wrong, you are right. By entering the magic door you've turned on the light so happiness is yours tonight for you're on your way to lite.

EXERCISE IS NOTHING: IT'S THE FAST
Excise Exercise!

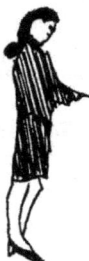

We are told to exercise but exercise pales in comparison to fasting in the release of HGH. Besides falling into our destiny, on a fast one can achieve a state of health that no form or amount of exercise could ever accomplish. Although exercise does increase HGH, with fasting and protein it's not necessary for superior health and maximum longevity. The implications of this fact and the contradiction from all we've been told cannot be overstated. With a fast your body and face grow younger right before your eyes! The rejuvenation of the skin is clearly visible as lines, wrinkles, blotches, and discolorations disappear reflecting the improvements within (now you won't show where you've been). No matter what you can take it on the chin and not show chagrin—just wear your fat-fastarian grin. Eat your cheese then don't eat, for if you want to be great it's a deadly sin.

FASTING LOWERS INSULIN RESISTANCE

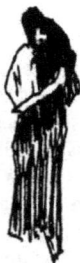

And when you do eat remember that insulin (from sugar and starch) inhibits HGH but fasting and protein lowers insulin resistance--so now insulin can't over-secrete and store fat as much. Daily fasting makes it possible for the insulin-resistant to eat fruit again--the carbohydrate level beyond which we store fat keeps changing and that sliding variable is initiated through the fast. Week-end fat-fasting is your sudden contrast so it negates the deadly hand of the past. Fruits only produce a modest rise in HGH so these are the only (limited) sugars to consume. Get wisdom here: fauna-fat and fruit brings youth and all else means doom. It's the high-sugar (starch) foods that create gloom but eat frugal fruit and you'll bloom. Follow this routine and you're wearing God's perfume but eat starch and grains and you're ready for a tomb.

JUST FOR THE WEEKEND: THE HIGHEST BLEND

ARTS OF PALEO FASTING

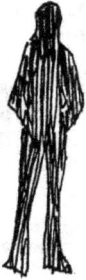

The easiest way to increase HGH is to eat protein then fast: the Sacred Sabbath Fast. The Bible says the Lord will "renew your youth as the eagle." I'm saying you must get regal: serene as a seagull and cute as a beagle. End this lull you've been in: stop sin, stick out your chin, love spiritual kin and now fast for this wonderful weekend—no more a has-been. Get ready for beautiful skin and the thin that's in. You'll wear our grin being as thin as a pin. Or fast after one meal a day and even "blue Mondays" become great (that's no spin). Remember our modern diet defers radically from our evolutionary past and God's design, so just one worthy weekender returns you to the ageless blueprint God designed for you alone. No more a mindless clone—you want to be shown and once you've flown you'll know what to do when the next time you groan. Whenever you're sore, open that magic door.

BACK FIVE UP TEN

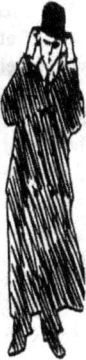

So you slipped? God turns all-bad to all-good for those who love the Lord. You can instantly come back twice as good as you were, then coals of ashes are heaped on the shamed ones who rose up against you in your weakness. We may slip but as champs we always come back stronger, much to everyone's surprise. From mud to roses: welcome to the real reality of regal right-brain living where you always win especially when you lose—for right then God swoops down to lift you to the mind cruise. This is fat-fasting! Fast to become a legend in your time. Your True Self rings like a chime so to the heights you can climb. To stay down is a crime as with God you'll make far more than a dime so in water just squeeze a lime. With fasting you're always at your prime: it's just a matter of cleaning out the slime, then you're sublime. This life must be your whole focus, not just part-time.

SACRED SABBATH FASTING:
Sleep

27

ARTS OF PALEO FASTING

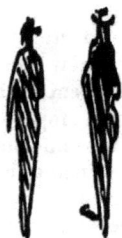

A good night's sleep is vitally important since it is during this time that most HGH is released. The body "grows" while we sleep, repairing and maintaining itself; and lack of soundness or duration decreases HGH—need I say any more about the incredible importance of a good night's sleep? Rest is religious: We must have part of the week where we think of nothing but God--that's the worthy week-ender Sacred Sabbath Fast. During this period you step into another reality all of your making. Once past the magic door you adapt to no one and thus it is sacred. Less food-messing, more mind-resting in the arms of God in a magic fairy land called eternity. Mine always start on Wednesdays when I enter into collapsed time, a gold mine.

ETERNAL CONSCIOUSNESS
The Fat Moment

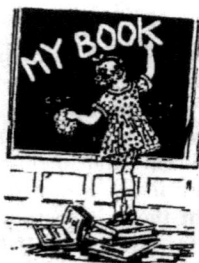

As a child I thought of nothing but my destiny. There is no greater joy than eternity: sitting in the magic moment where past, present and future unite. Practice with me today: as you appreciate this Friday think of all the Fridays of your entire life. Remember how you felt as a kid excited about going to the movies or in anticipation of the week-end. Think of all the cloudy Fridays if it's cloudy or all the blue-skied Fridays if its sunny. The more eternal your consciousness the healthier you are. Especially if living in nature this collapsed time can create deep thought for hours or days in what is called the "fertile anarchy" of genius leading to discovery. Here is your full recovery: fast and wait for instructions. When God speaks obey immediately. Do not procrastinate—skillfully navigate the tides of nature: when the rain falls, success sprouts! Just fast and be ready for your reward—you'll never again be bored.

ETERNAL WEEK-END

ARTS OF PALEO FASTING

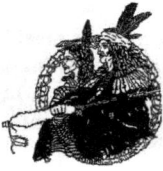

Fasting is the way to humility, bringing all-power: "Because he stooped so low God has exalted him." Humble yourself, for humility precedes riches and honor. For the sacred week-ender , shift gears entirely. If music is a powerful force play something different for the whole time period. It's important that you "step into" another world, another reality transcending all time and space. Stay eternal, that's the kernel--the unique seed symbol at birth which contains all of your potentials. It's the truths in you which comes out: those are your credentials and these are the essentials.

THE INNER LIFE IS ALL

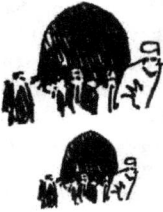

On this sacred week-end you'll find the inner life far more important than the outer one. This inner life is our reputation with God, the only source of blessings. The outer life is our rep with people—but fame is fleeting and infamy occurs with just one meeting. Never trust the vicissitudes of human nature and public opinion. Go inside, ride the tide with nothing to hide. You'll feel such pride after going inside and on this high tide you'll glide with God as your guide. Forget all from the outside--just for the week-end set all else aside for you're about to go worldwide. It's in heaven you'll reside once the world you've denied. So fast with pride: you'll be the superior man or woman bonafide. Once you've complied you'll be over-supplied for your future is so wide as God promises to provide. He knows how you cried but now all that has died through the fast which you'll have tried. It's only with the outer world you did collide.

DIGESTIVE, ASSIMILATIVE, ELIMINATIVE

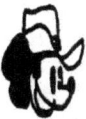

Here's the "full" reason for fasting to stay hyper-creative everlasting: There are three food systems: digestive, assimilative and eliminative. 85% of all our energy goes into one of the three and all this energy is released when fasting. But if "stuck" in the digestive system all day not only do we lack that energy but the assimilative and eliminative gets dull—everything goes into a lull. Just skip dinner: fasting all afternoon gives the elimination time to work for full evacuation in the morning. This is a warning to avoid the next day's mourning.

ARTS OF PALEO FASTING

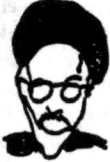

Ramadan fasters may over-eat starch in the early Suhuur meal in apprehension of the day's fast. In elevating insulin, by night they're famished and overeat again (how you can you sleep, my friend?). But with fat you not only look and feel so good all day the fast elevates more ketones so hunger diminishes even more. Don't follow the crowd--they haven't a clue as through the herd anti-fat dogma (so loud) the facts they misconstrue. But you'll now daily renew with all things anew. Fast as long as you can between meals and eat only when hungry. Without this discipline you'll be uptight even angry.

COOK WITH THE GANG

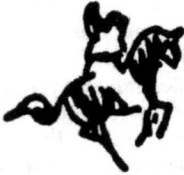

Cooking and eating excites them to run to the fun, then blues has begun. Cook with the gang? They'll all want to hang. Food's got tang like a big bang but as the devil's fang you'll feel it in pangs. I'll tell you the truth: it'll ruin your tooth. Like the Indians: can you see how the chips make the holes? Corn takes its tolls. Be thin like poles-(no rolls): it's good for your souls. Don't give up your goals just to eat: give up the wheat then watch who you meet. Sickness you'll cheat as fortune you'll greet. Fast is turning up the heat as you enter the world-beat. Even if eating meat things will stay neat so you may compete with all work complete. Life will stay sweet if just fruit or fat is your treat so now join our ELITE. It's like taking a retreat to the devil's defeat--the bad will excrete while your bank roll's replete.

THEY WEAR A SPARE TIRE
Staying Lean vs. Getting Mean

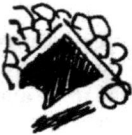

Obesity shuts down HGH then depression takes over. There is a perfect correlation between body fat percentage and blocked HGH. Obesity shuts it down since fat is a food reserve and HGH is secreted from depletion of that reserve (fasting). I'm no liar—they wear a spare tire. Am I wrong? Look at the throng. As they walk they mock their Maker and the blueprint design of perfection-to-be. Fast: to be at your best after your rest--then you'll be blessed. You've passed the test and the reward is being filled with zest. I can attest: in refusing to digest I was no more stressed nor depressed. So I say rest

30

before rule while you fast to the last. There is no past so let it all dissolve as you resolve all riddles, rid of all meddlers.

BREAKFAST-ONLY PLAN

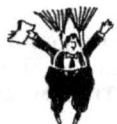

Most people prefer to skip breakfast and eat lunch or dinner and that's fine. But many see breakfast as the most important meal of the day and as the only meal that's ok. I've always loved the breakfast-only plan, for now that you have your daily meal *behind* you that's it—there's no more eating for the day. This acts as an incredible safety-net for compulsive eaters. For they're now fasting, they're not hungry and not thinking about food (the crude). I call this the "psychology of having the meal behind thee plan". That settles it in mind as the warrior sticks to his decision and the day remains blissful with no thoughts of food. If you break down in the afternoon have a little cheese or raw milk which carries you through the day. In the fasting state you have a right to a siesta for only "if one eats must he work." Eat all day, you stay a clerk (the eater seeking approval with a smirk). Through the fast this worldly chaos you shirk and your energy shoots up: you're about to perk. But the eater gets selfish (he becomes a jerk as his quirks go berserk). But if you don't eat you have a right not to work but just to sleep. From the bad past you won't hear a peep and you'll start to ascend—it will be *sudden, and steep.*

LET THE PRISONERS GO FREE
You've Found Gold—No Longer "Old"

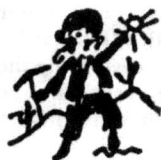

Eat, then put it away. Sleep all day if you must for after today your life will have changed—it's all been arranged. From food we deranged and from God we estranged but with the fast we de-caged and then found our True Selves never aged. Now go on to destiny to never again be upstaged--for the glories ahead you've never even waged. All your problems are gone as you banish the bad associations with whom you're engaged. Remember how they enraged, how on your properties they rampaged? Through the fast you've disengaged so now you're body, mind and spirit is assuaged.

ARTS OF PALEO FASTING

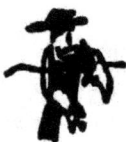

Regarding those dark phases of our life when filled with strife: It's been shown that fasting and zero-carb dieting cures even schizophrenia—we've been given a free fail-free device to be free of fear and the old age madness of King Lear. Fear and confusion leaves the faster fast and that's why it's a blast. That poor identity (caste) will not last—it's all in the past, yet the future's so vast. And that flesh you amassed? Just wait and see the contrast. What of the foes who harassed and then so miscast? Them we'll outlast for now we're unsurpassed.

NO MORE A SICK THICK--JUST SLICK
No Hunger? It's a Call to Fast

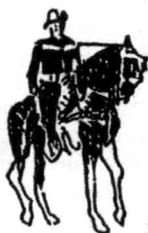

If you have no hunger it's God's call to fast and embark on this futuristic (yet old-world) phantasmagoria so vast. If suffering the proclivities of cruel human nature it's a call to fast, for then it won't last—you'll have overcome how they miscast. If you heed that call by just drinking distilled water with lemon you'll sail effortlessly through this blissful time (with class). Every time I did this something very important occurred for which I was totally ready: in my prime, ready for the climb with just water and lime. We must kill the flesh to get to the power of the spirit behind it. Ignore any stomach pain for it's just cleansing of the most clogged organ (the sewer main). Once clean the hunger's gone and you'll have Einstein's brain. Now for the power of a queen: the degree of gut-encumbrance determines your looks (your sheen). Remember this slogan: no more thick and sick but slick (like you've never seen). The would-be queen should always remember that every time she denies hunger pain (refuses to give in) the face becomes more beautiful. For the reasons above you're pulled up into the shape of a dove so soon you'll attract love.

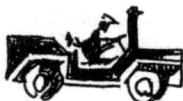

If one is dealing with old sludge (from years of eating fudge) the fast can be quite uncomfortable, the looks terrible. That's why Ramadan Fasting makes so much sense: Eat fat in the morning then you're not hungry the whole glorious fasting day. Then at night when you're hungry again take piece cheese or fruit to eliminate all residue. I say a few for too much sugar inhibits HGH in bed so for some of you perhaps a bite of cheese instead. Take one bite

ARTS OF PALEO FASTING

then just sit tight (that's true might: doing things right). Since calorie restriction also releases human growth hormone just eating less works incredibly well--that way you're continuously fasting by eating mouse-meals of raisons or fat then going right back into the fast. Go austere: your (new) time is near.

FASTING MIRACLES SABBATICAL

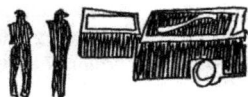

When things approach critical mass: to the world just go dead and take a fasting miracles sabbatical instead—a period of great contemplation when you do nothing but fast and think. Day one will evince a great miracle and day two an even greater one: These "magic coincidences" only come from God so avenge not yourself--let God overcome the clod. There is no one to call or see, nothing to do--just fast and the success-source arrives in full view (he who God has chosen will mysteriously come forth too). Just retreat into your inner world: Fasting works every time by intention alone, then all your dreams come true.

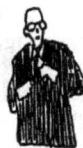

If you don't want ZERO-CARB try the alternative Grape Cure: For three days take only 1/3 cup raisins spread throughout the day. The gut will shrink to a walnut, the balance regained and your whole life will have changed. What a relief for the thinner you are the less you'll eat and the more fast, quick, ecstatic, creative and spiritual you will get (it's so sweet). Suddenly you become a hail-fellow-well-met (for fasting is just eating less) so you'll be on top free of fret—the best bet. It's just like an old table restored to reveal the beautiful rosewood underneath—just one short fast and you'll be floating like a beautiful leaf, though still the chief. Fasting is the only way to end all grief for anti-depressants just dull (or kill)— any true happiness is brief but fasting brings true relief.

FAST FOR MAXIMUM DIGESTION

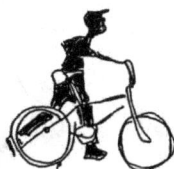

After fasting for an entire day—like from breakfast-to-breakfast—one can hardly imagine the delights of digestion, assimilation and elimination. Fasting is the way to "wake-up" the entire system and make it work maximally. How to have super-health: rest the whole works. Fast: don't delay, do it today and you'll see an array: of people, places and things attracted in at your will (ending the foray). This new life will surely fill the bill as no more you'll get the cold chill. The painful past was just a drill to show the results of lust (from eating your fill). So now you'll enjoy the good life of fasting (even after the grill)! The medical recommendations of grains and corn (not fat) paleo science has made life nil—the dry skin, wrinkles and endless hunger were like sinking in swill! It all made you ill putting you through the mill—it was hard swallowing that pill from fat-phobic culture making you dull, dead, bored (it was a brain-kill). You've got skill and it now out-spills as the old life goes still. It'll be such a thrill as destiny fulfills so look to the horizon—will you be going to Brazil? The best of all: *the look, the feel, the experience--and never again being ill.*

THE 24-HOUR MINI-FAST

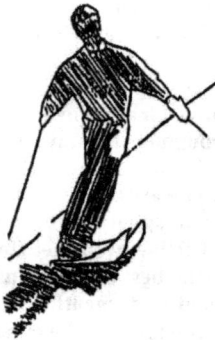

The first day of the mini-fast (from breakfast-to-breakfast, lunch-to-lunch) may be difficult. Just know that each day it gets easier and more rewarding. Every time you do it you'll feel better than the day before as the benefits accrue. With each meal digestion is quicker and more exhilarating, assimilation more penetrating and elimination more automatic. This defines real vibrant health--true wealth. I mean svelte: they'll melt as you walk-in, no more mocking because now you're a-rocking. I'm talking: just aspire to the higher (out of the mire) becoming a live-wire: thin, flexible and also mentally independent—that's so fine, no more towing their line. You're a gold-mine yet so kind! The old constipation made you blind for it's not the fats or fruits that bind—it's all those grains you've left behind. Now you'll be refined for it's the superior man's find. After your heavenly week-end you'll have a brilliant mind for the fast is the best rest—a way to unwind but with total industry combined. The old obstructions it will now confine for it was you they maligned (that's the way of mankind). But with the fast, foes have no effect if its with the stars, sun and moon you're entwined.

DOWN WITH FRUIT-GLUTTONY
Up with Fat-Fasting Bliss

ARTS OF PALEO FASTING

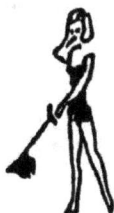

Years ago I felt fat and had had it: I decided to fast and end all my troubles. Throughout the day I could actually feel the fat melting down--I was getting thinner and quicker and this lightness brought elation. It became an addiction and I was thin from that point until: I read about fruitarianism and instead of fasting I got into gluttonous fruit-eating (even though Ehret condemned it). Constant fruit-eating ruined my life until I returned to dairy fat then fast for the day. I was exhilarated with a creative phantasmagoria and began to say "down with continuous fruit-eating and up with fat-fasting bliss!" It's a wonderful feeling God's kiss so don't eat lest you miss this and fall back into abyss. That eating life made you miss (you felt it was all that exist because it's like a snake charmer: hunger's a his). So no more remiss and with such a beautiful future you'll lose all need to reminisce.

SACRIFICIAL FAST AND REST

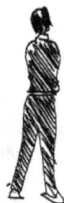

Decide in the morning whether today is a Ramadan (day) or Buddha (afternoon) fast then do it just that way. It's your actions backed with intention creating strength and character so say "my Sabbath rest starts now". Despite this period of "spiritual leisure" most "business" (underground work and creative action) occurs here and it's as good as it gets. How to make it big: leave maximum time for God the Giver of all things (especially the impossible) and get ready for your jets.

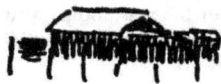

To sacrifice and seclude removes the feud and improves your mood. Word and faith preachers ask for donations: The more we give the more we receive. The fast works on the same principal of ten-fold increase. God doesn't need our money---He reads our *sacrifices* based on faith, and fasting is the biggest sacrifice! Deprive your gut, God removes the rut. Give a "fast offering"--fast for seven lunches a week then give the money you saved give away (the increase will flow in that day). More than investments there is no bigger pay. Timing is all in God's Kingdom but the fast is the catalyst for everything on your list. To overcome obstruction is the highest form of prayer (confronting the devil's hiss) so as you fast and release HGH you won't be "doing" anything yet nothing's left amiss! "Rest before rule" is another way of saying "exhaustion precedes completion". You're now going to

ARTS OF PALEO FASTING

fast to let the Highest fight your battles (this is the gist): Just stop-eating, pray
and rely on God's fist. For only God knows the future so whenever tired just
rest and recoup in bed, for only He knows what lies ahead.

FAST-REPENT FOR GOD'S REVENGE

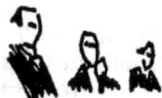

You must always see how much your exhaustion comes from
oppression—letting inferiors in to rain on your parade (you
get jade) and take the wind out of your sails (God heard your
wails). For example, do you have backstabbing, belittling
relatives? Get ready for the big payback: soon you'll see it as fact for God's
revenge is necessary for the relief of the Saints as proof that God is just (He's
firm but has tact) and to think otherwise brings aging cynicism—you
rust. Those sting-shots and flip-flops brought constant stress as recurrently
your joys did combust. Abuse gave you thorns as it formed an ugly crust but
fast-repentance dissolves this induced-schizophrenia from others (distorted
implants and templates) which blocked success through self-disgust. Recall
always our slogan: All men are sinners (your accusers are filled with lusts)!

PRESTO, YOU'RE BACK ON TOP

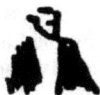

Whenever you feel sad, rejected, constricted, bloated and in need
of toning--a fat-fast is indicated. As weekends are for eating out
and since low-carb gives you clout the two-speed week's the best
route.   See the body streamline as all bloat goes out.   Moods,
emotions, mentality, physicality, spirituality become even so just for the week-
end keep carbs below 15 and you'll have something to believe in. The result is
abundance, joy and getting thin so you'll say "I've never been so happy since
I don't remember when." To enter this new life, just begin: stop eating and go
within—by your mere decision the past is gone along with all chagrin.

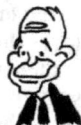

Fat-Fast for the Sacred Sabbath Week-end. You'll see how little you
need once ketosis gets rolling. While you're bowling you won't hear
stomach growling and you'll be happy just strolling. Say "No" to
their cajoling to eat wrong or you'll need consoling. Not controlling
what you eat   (giving in to sweet or wheat)   makes puffy thy
seat. We're talking how to compete (not take a back seat nor suffer defeat) for
now you're the elite. So let me repeat: take a retreat *then* conquer Wall
Street. It's all that chaos you'll   beat then old age and disease you'll

ARTS OF PALEO FASTING

cheat. Though simple it's a major feat while also being a delightful treat. Your work is sure to complete while destiny you'll greet—see all those food demons rushing out as a fleet? Now heal all you meet while remaining discreet. After the glorious fat-of-the-land weekend expect something magnificent to happen on Monday: welcome to God's Buffet. Now no more stray from the fast or it's back to dismay, and let the past stay gone lest the future decay. This truth I convey will become as child's play, so today just enjoy the ray and pray to stay on top (not the bottom as prey).

FAT-FASTING IS TO FLOAT

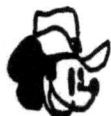

After many years of fruit-gluttony with no fasting I gave up that life of failure to thrive in pursuit of a much higher creative life of OMMAD: One Meat Meal a Day. So many think elimination won't work with fats—"they're binding"--but nothing is further from the truth. Since the colon needs fat to operate you'll say "it's a wonderful new find" as your maximum evacuations end the old grind. As everyday it all eliminates you'll be never angry but kind, and see how dark depression comes from constipation making you sad and blind. This food-life is ideal--it's the real deal and it's unbelievable how you'll feel, like floating on wheels and winning mass appeal. Just try it: see what glory reveals. You'll be so appetite-suppressed you'll keep postponing your meals. This truly is the life, as fat electrically conducts spirit for real magnetism and shining like steel.

TINY MOUSE-MEALS MAKE SHOW-STEALS
Listen: All She-Hulks and Family Terrorists

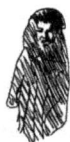

Come out of your shell now. The HQ (Higher Quality) food is far more calorie-dense, the determinant of food quality. This potent HQ requires far less bulk to release energy to the encephalization (enlargement) of the brain—the beautiful elongation of the head. Overdoing the HQ is missing the point--we wish to shrink the gut while enlarging the brain. It's like pulling God's chain with so much to gain. And what did you give up: it was only the grain and large meals (as main). You need only to fast and this is nothing you can feign. With the fat-fast you're rid of all pain and it didn't even feel like you abstained. You've so much more to attain so make it a giant campaign and no more complain.

ARTS OF PALEO FASTING

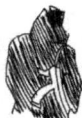

That old life was so inane but now with the fast it's greatness to maintain while being rid of that sordid old life (so mundane). So let me instruct so health will sustain and then how to reign. I'll make it plain: The food devil in you must stay slain--the only way of staying sane. It's really insane how it left such a serious stain: on your nerves and looks it was a strain as that crud went through your veins. But now with the fauna fast the upward-energy and creativity is so much better than cocaine as energy you can hardly contain! A little more if I may explain: the bad in your food behavior and associations you must continue to disdain. From those old sins and systems you must completely refrain if in this new joy you plan to remain. The difference between good and the bad you must always ascertain so the good life you can retain. As your fruit and fat needs are met you'll reach natural thinness (which you'll surely attain).

FIND THE LINE: SHINE AND SWELL

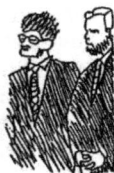

You must find the line between *shine* and *swell*. The HQ is so potently powerful you'll need little for the shine but more may swell. Find that line and never be fat again: As you get as thin as tin you'll become hyper-sensitive and see how food makes the brain spin. During this fasting process just bite the bullet and begin. You may want to eat to stop the fasting (withdrawal) process so see it as sin and if you eat just start the fast again. But I'm encouraging you to go through the fire: garnishing self-control will make you a rod of power with assured success soon (your foes will cower). If you shine without swell you'll stand as tall as a tower—that's how you'll reign so don't cave in (keep regal power). This change with you on top (for once) puts you above criticism which used to fall like a shower.

ONE DAILY FAT DOSAGE

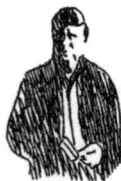

Fat-eating should be localized into the one meal. Eat to your satisfaction. Just eat fat in the morning or fruit (I wouldn't) then fat for lunch then fast to the next day. Unless one is fat-fasting (no fructose) eating fat more than once can be counterproductive. You only need one "daily dosage" of (one exposure to) the fabulous fat--although there are people who eat a "thumb size" of cheese every couple hours with great success. Find your perfect fit for fat-curtailment becomes an exact science.

ARTS OF PALEO FASTING

As overdoing fat is easy I suggest the following routine: awake and have your morning drink to release the bowels and wait as long as you can to indulge, then fast—while expecting miracles from God who will always reward with the new day's blast.

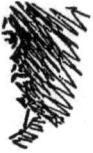

Expect life-changing events from anywhere at any time, so just look forward with expectancy and glee as you enjoy your water and lime. On a fast God said "clasp your hand in Mine and lose not thine hold. For you can't tell the great things I have for thee through the smallest happening. Thine every hair is numbered and I delight in taking the most incidental occurrences to reveal my earnestness in helping thee. Look not back but ahead to the glory I have prepared for thee." This thrilled my soul as I sat in eternity. I want this for you too--and it's all for free.

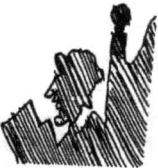

To be receptive to this miracle you must be properly-fueled and empty with the energy in the head. So the fat-fasting program is both about fasting and eating the correct food. For most people coming off the SAD diet fat is necessary methadone as the toxins flood the bloodstream. It's a delicious transition keeping them stable and receptive when fasting as diets are switched. The point is to stick to higher paleo and fast in between for the result of eating wrong is one depressed mood (no sheen). I don't want be crude but eating that other way made you one ugly dude as with mates you would feud, to the TV you were glued and ever in a bad mood (let alone how you looked in the nude). Did your friends call you "rude" when in emotions you stewed, or from porn you viewed (since you stayed un-renewed)? But now these problems the fast has preclude and now you're accomplishing the dreams you've pursued. Do you remember coming unglued as everything you said they misconstrued? Now I conclude: if the fast you include it's a wonderful aroma you'll exude as with God you're imbued and success will no longer allude.

CARBOHYDRATE LEVEL OF WEIGHT GAIN

ARTS OF PALEO FASTING

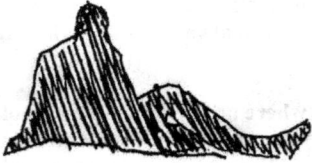

The carbohydrate level beyond which one gains weight is raised through lowcarb dieting and fasting. As a result after the week-end fat-fast insulin-sensitivity is regained and *some* can again eat fruit. You will love the frugal fruit and fat routine. If in fasting one becomes hungry just a few raisons eliminates the mucus causing the pain. You're now doing the grape cure—you've switched from fasting to one of the greatest cures on earth. Keep to this, don't add more and return to the fast--the "gut fixed". Isn't it wonderful to rewrite the script? Into God's paint you've been dipped away from the old life in which you were gripped. If on your shoulder it was chipped it's now from off your back the monkey's been ripped as to hell the demons are shipped: your problems have been whipped. They made you ugly: so nondescript but with God you're entirely equipped as the foe's been outstripped.

FOOD DARKENS THE AURA

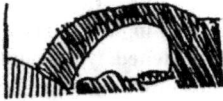

Do something different this week-end: Fast and look forward to a brand new life Monday. You don't have to seek spas or the clutter in health food stores. Just make this week-end a luxurious "coming out" party in preparation for your new life from just two days filled with your achievement of excessive Human Growth Hormone. I'll tell you my scheme (it's the same old theme): I'm not the type mean but we have to get lean. No more the bean and you'll get the sheen, that is: clean. It's not all your gene: just fast to be keen, that's our scene. Look like a teen—that's when you wean off the burrito: though it raises libido you'll lose in casino, look bad in tuxedo. Food darkens the aura not like the glamorous Zorro but a pest like bandito or mosquito.

DISABLING UGLY/FAT GENES

ARTS OF PALEO FASTING

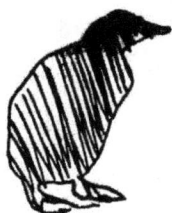

No more excuses for it's just you who loses: It's the devil who accuses but God rewards all who rightly chooses. Yes ugliness and obesity is genetic if you eat like your ancestors and family members. But if you go FFF you'll disable the thrifty gene (which holds on to fat and calories) and all other gene-codes choking your sheen. As your whole family is fat, you'll resemble a teen and as they are dumb, you'll be keen. I tell you truly it's the wrong (culturally-induced, raw vegan-seduced, low-fat deduced) diet encouraged by constant advertising and deluded doctor-produced dogma that has distorted your looks. You can separate from the kooks and the boring vegan cooks: just eat what you really want: the most delicious (to humans, dogs and cats) _saturated animal fat_—and ignore the thousands of vegan books. Now you'll have movie-star looks without supporting the "health store" crooks.

It's most important that you stop everything and just look out the window now. Let God fill it all in, wow!

HAPPY FAT-FAST

Higher Paleo-Fasting Calms Anorexic Emotions
from the "Burning Building Syndrome"

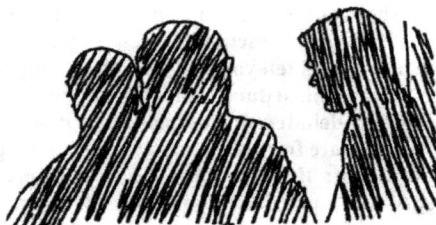

"LIFE IS HELL"

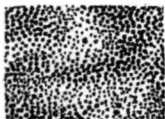

The anorexic says : "life is hell—pure chaos surrounds me. The only thing that soothes and activates in spite of it all is fasting." Could this be true? Bible Christians of old fasted all the time, in the face of good or bad—for celebration or help in times of trouble. It is only in our modern Dionysian pleasure-loving obese generation that the art of fasting has been lost. The tendency to fast at any and all situations is in all major and native religions. So is the anorexic crazy? Or is she cosmic with an aesthetic ingrown understanding of a basic truth innate to the animal kingdom? In my past I was surrounded by harassing Hitlerian harridans and a degrading matrix where I was viewed as a contemptible "nothing". I survived it by sequestering myself in the smallest room in the house with my cat who was my only friend. I had gut-pain and fear from a young age but overcoming these conspiracies I became a sage. I had to fast to not succumb to inner rage: only through fasting could I escape this cage. I lived to tell the story so here it starts for all of you stuck backstage. Are you ready for your new age? You must disengage from old systems and habits holding you down--then your pain will assuage and you'll get a celebrity's wage.

MODERN SOCIETY CHAOS

ARTS OF PALEO FASTING

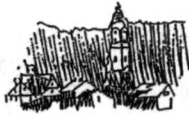

Much of this treatise about "ana" is a hypersensitive cerebrotonic's reaction to chaos living in human society. Am I pro-ana? No I am pro-fasting and understand anorexia well enough to know we must magnify this good "ana" trait and squash the deadly ones which are *maladaptations to chaos*. Anorexia turns deadly when a sense of God is lost, when she sees her own control as the only answer to what she senses as "dirty disorder". Yes there is chaos, but God's help is the only way out and fasting is God's instruction to the saints to get to that peaceful power. Until we use this key our lives remain dead, our genius dormant. It's a special instruction for special people for it is fasting which brings success and prosperity--not meaningless assiduity, Godless perfectionism and sinking in our own swill of binging, purging and alcohol relapse. Due to the explosion of videos across the world every country shows an epidemic of anorexia--women seek the thin (for to men it's "in"). Whereas they used to love the curvaceous and voluptuous, now it's anorexic thin-lass fuss—weighing less is a must. Anorexia the disease is a mess—we want to be ANA, the mature recovered anorexic beauty (not excess, which is lack of progress). If you be ana you'll always have those characteristics into middle age: love of privacy, God and the inner journey. That's your new address as to God through the fast you'll always have access. You must separate the real disease from the superior characteristics (mislabeled as "disease") that will bring you ease.

BURNING BUILDING SYNDROME
The Intense Anorexogenic System Happens to Males Too

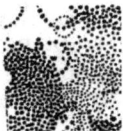

It's like peaceful serenity vs. wartime: the system becomes blocked. One can surely see why the anorexic would have this syndrome, for look at her complex: being born in the anorexogenic system (i.e. the system to which anorexia is an appropriate reaction) where the striving to "be" was obstructed: it's a sexist system which disconfirms her. (If the ana be a male it's still a stultifying system with a terrifying male authority—all these set-ups relate to males too). In this set-up she knows that whatever she thinks/wants/feels has no effect on the outer system—she has absolutely no control over her circumstances or how they see her. In any disconfirming system the victim's actions do not change the projected image. Now the whole sense of efficacy is "shifted" from the interpersonal scenario to the intrapsychic sphere where she controls her own inner world and body. This sense of outer powerlessness brings fear, transformed to self-control and thus starts the syndrome of the

43

ARTS OF PALEO FASTING

overachieving but completely isolated soul. Whenever the fear (feeling of utter powerlessness) erupts, ana fasts or feasts. But by shifting to the fruit and fat-fast emotions will be soothed, skin is smoothed and the personality cooled. For the hospitalized ana, if she wishes to be fruitarian then temporarily avocado with acid fruit once a day for the major meal will also bring her life into total order—this she desperately needs, for eating disorders automatically create the sense of catastrophic chaos. That's why anorexia is now called "DE": disordered eating, which for the Ana is heaven-cheating while success is fleeting.

THE PROJECTION OF FROGS
Instantaneous Conflict

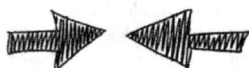

Adding to her helpless position she's in the land of mesomorphic "bigs"—control freaks who disrespect this otherworldly inward creature: this weak meek thing. If she's lucky she gets to know God: As His child she knows she's great when she fasts, staying mild. But the world doesn't see her that way: her fasting may bring hospitalization, and before she matures into a dignified lady with high boundaries taking full control of her own domain she's sunk—having to adapt to other people who see her as junk, an upstart punk avoided like a skunk. For the mesomorphs with the somatomic personality (of social, dominance, control) are incapable of understanding the ectomorph of cerebrotonic temperament (privacy, inward, spiritual). (For a perfect rendition of the interactional condition see Streetcar Named Desire). To her it seems like frogs and hogs lording it over her with stupid cruelty and angry niceties. To avoid fearful anxiety she's learned to have nothing on her stomach to "stay high" as the only way to escape/overcome disaster in this volatile context. But when she fasts she's incarcerated against her will. The anorexic may not exist to those around her as she's treated like a "thing" or a "disease" (being a projection is a scary thing).

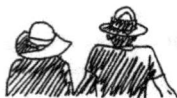

When I was in this position, until I learned to fast daily life became overwhelming and even eating the right food was too much. One day I got a flat tire. No one in town wanted to fix it—it was "just a bike" so I tried everything to no avail for I had no control of the outer world—everyone turned their back. I started to fast and everything suddenly worked out. From so many like situations the anorexic comes to know this fact and begins to feel that fasting is her destiny—putting her in synchronicity—and to not do so creates chaos. In this

44

extraordinary life the fast works in fact, releasing all blocks. As the eater who eats at frustration loses every time, the ana-faster fasts at it with water and lime (or goes beyond the problem to the sublime),

LETTER TO HAPPY FAT-FASTARIANS:
Arise: They Won't Despise and You'll Take the Prize

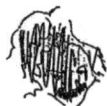

We're a nation guarding our food ration. Urination—with lots of distilled lemonade—deletes the toxins maintaining our lower station. Let's face it: our inclination keeps us bitterly separated, a lonely corporation while we could be the epitome of God's Creation, a divine formation. Are you ready to take the throne as an emerging foundation? Let's fast as a vacation—wow, what a sensation! Are you ready for flotation like ascending to a space station? I tell you truthfully all else (for us) is stagnation. This isn't self-starvation (for that is psychotic sedation) but rather fighting temptation as our sanity salvation. Our life's been on probation with little or no relation (what a mess) but now having overcome the aberration we're just fastarians getting total admiration and no more accusation. Fast and you'll delight in your coloration and in you life's work the culmination (it's a real coronation).

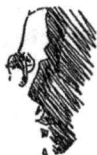

With many of you I've had a lovely conversation. Before we became a nation it was giant constipation—of thought, work and love--but now we've got the right combination to become great stars in the congregation. We're known for our animation--superiority through aviation. To get there we eat right to improve our location (like a hierarchy gradation) and it's due to our fasting-elation. Are you fasting? Then receive God's carnation, a work and success-causation. The barf-cessation stopped our impending cremation and looking like a crustacean (bulimia was ego and life-deflation). Just being a lady will now trigger a big donation for all else is frustration and joy-negation. Are you ready to reach you life's aspiration? Then to the bad there must be amputation for your life must be holy (it's a matter of vibration). Are you ready to make fasting your vocation? It's ok if it's fixation--if it's for God revelation and fulfilled expectation.

ARTS OF PALEO FASTING

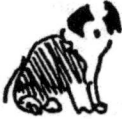

[Why I ended up with a managerie]: Now about your blood relation. There's been a severe altercation--I know the pitfalls of that association for it's hard to forget the aggravation and agitation from dis-association. But rid of my disease I have only adoration and free-flow expression (i.e. unobstructed oration). It's the realization after the hellish life before the saint's full inspiration. But the ladylike fast is total transformation--almost a gene-mutation. Being sick I was mis-creation (hating the self through mutilation) ending in dehydration then hospitalization. To my image it meant defamation--hardly a cute decoration when showing this deformation. And to my mind it meant desolation, desperation, a very bad reputation (seeming to them like retardation): despite my protestation all-good saw termination. Anorexia is mere vegetation--a tragic demonstration of destiny-obfuscation.

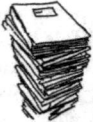

Well I prefer the limelight and worthy occupation. Life now has fascination, high motivation, happy exploration, healthy sanitation and divine dedication. With grape-aid my libation I soar as all systems experience dilation. Now I have conjugation and it's like a giant federation—we're a new ana-generation. In all life's cycles we show skillful navigation and through all life's duration we're happy stars like a constellation. Without reservation you must fast: this is full relaxation and for me it finally meant publication. It's so much fun the body-mysticism from fasting, like elongation (and what fascination)! Just taking a walk is a wonderful education and the means of divination. After the fast it's time for celebration.

SOLUTION: FAT-FASTING BLISS

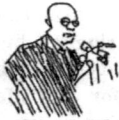

"It feels like World War". Anorexics suffer from the "burning building syndrome" like trying to escape a burning building with no exit. It never ends--this sense of terrifying chaos--so they seek food (mother's love) for release, but then the chaos just increased. The anorexic is in a WAR (many watch documentaries on WWII just so they can relate to something they understand). When in this state try fat-fasting: cutting out all fruit sugar and living on tomavo, doughless pizza or Red Salad. Some of you may prefer a brazil or macadamia nut or for lacto-fruitarians a sliver of cheese when hungry. Free of sugar your emotions will be soothed and the hormone glucagons will be elevated from the fat, bringing a comforting state of fat-burning, a release of retained water (adding pressure) and calming of the emotions.

ARTS OF PALEO FASTING

KK BIOGRAPHY
Chaos Leads to New Psych Theory

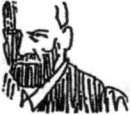

From all this pressure I developed a new theory in psychology, as major as Freud, Bateson and Jung. I had always been so much in this state of felt chaos I had to leave civilization and live alone in the desert wilderness. I felt minimized in groups as if I didn't exist while feeling their meanest projections. I had to escape not only the system but society as a whole, then I had to fast. For mentally and emotionally I was still stuck and each day was torture. Feeling controlled by people was a constant strangulation and so in my twenties childhood complexes and fears (along with leaving home for the first time) manifested in fullblown anorexia. It was terrible, compulsive, subconscious, desperate. This is how this theory included food problems: At age 30 I "found" Ehretism and fruitarianism but being impatient to become "fruitarian" I bypassed the transit diet and got right into fruit-gluttony and the result was dissolved teeth and hyper-insulinism along with uncontrollable mood swings and anger. When I found Atkins I fat-fasted for one year on just one meal a day of cheese omelet. I stabilized then craved fruit with cheese: lacto-fruitarianism was the end and the new beginning. This high-tech combo gave me the high-speed consciousness of ethereal miracles I craved so I stabilized with fruit, reversing into fat-fasting whenever I felt bloated, constricted, dry, chapped, agitated or stuporus. The skin system revived instantly along with the nerves. The *fat-fast was my trump card* for within a short time I was normal again and could return to sweet fruit and fasting. Now I could relax and work on my bad associations and habits.

ANOREXIC SYMPTOMS
Fat-Fasting the First Step to Spirituality

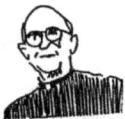

I had spiritual cravings and joined every church who left me in the lurch. I then concentrated on my own inner journey combined with eating right: fat-fasting with a little fruit at times. They're will be many gainsayers against the use of fat but most anorexics will agree there is no other way to meet our rare needs of order, simplicity, higher consciousness and beauty, emotional stability and the ability—once having eaten a satisfying meal—of fasting for long periods. I have found that the terrible symptoms of anorexia (magnified when bulimia is present) were eradicated by deleting all sugar and just eating low-carb

ARTS OF PALEO FASTING

fat. They are: (1) respiratory: paralysis, shortness of breath, asthmatic or difficult labored breathing and excessive coughing. (2) skin: desquamation (peeling in scales), dry, wrinkled, brittle and severely dehydrated skin, mineral loss, itchy skin, rashes and dryness covered with downy fuzz. (3) uglies: facial swelling, puffy or splotched face. (4) osteoporosis, shrunken bones, brittle splitting nails and wasted muscles. (5) digestive: mal-absorption syndrome, abdominal-bloating and acid pain. (6) fainting spells and blurred vision. (7) social isolation and occasional relapses into alcohol and drugs.

FAT AND THE COLON
Elimination Au Naturale

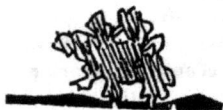

It has been found that the colon needs fat to operate perfectly. The best thing about this higher paleo diet is the supreme regularity and ease of evacuation like clockwork each morning. The roughage and fiber in fruit combined with the fat brings this daily relief which is the most important thing (since all recovery is elimination). Anas are constipated either from eating the wrong foods, bulimia, worry and emotions or not eating at the right times. But no more as the birdlike engine eats mouse-meals of cleansing fruit and colon-friendly fat and is instantly relieved. It's no chore for now each morning she's clean to the core. This wonderful new pattern opens the magic door—to this new day with opportunities and fun galore.

FAT-FASTING BRINGS ORDER

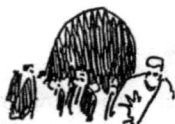

A man from France said of the fat-fast: " It's working so well it's a surprise to me and everyone else as I have lost twenty pounds. I have difficulties believing such changes as my energy level is astonishing. I feel so good--whether it's from the deletion of all sugar and starch or the addition of fruit fat I don't know but thanks for taking a chance by spreading a pro-fat theory helping people like me. I could never make it on just juicy fruit." Another lady said "I don't want to cook and have salads and spuds. I just want simplicity like a piece of cheese and later fresh fruit foods, a small meal after which I can easily fast for the day." Fear of fat or fat-phobia is cultural—cheese is basic to the beautiful Italians! People will not eat even avocado out of fear of fat so instead eat bread, crackers, sandwiches--and get

48

ARTS OF PALEO FASTING

fat just like that. Yet fruitarians who eat upwards to six avocados a day are bone thin (however I was still hungry—only animal fat filled the bill). Inferior foods build unsightly fat flesh while fat builds beautiful moist tissue. Eat fat, be happy and thin--and then fast.

SMOOTH SAILING
Fat-Fasting: Now True Leisure Begins

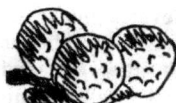

Leisure is the answer for anas, for creative answers and wit. But the anti-fat myth obstructs this: There is no bigger mantra in all health science as it seems a "self-evident fact". In the case of anorexics—birdlike engines who do best on the fast after eating small amounts of appetite-suppressing foods like fat--it is a dangerous falsehood. For if they avoid fat they must eat starch: then insulin perks appetite, fat is laid on (their phobia) and water is retained causing hypertension. These changes brought on by insulin are uncomfortable to most but excruciating to the birdlike ectomorph who is basically emotional, sensitive, socially mis-fitting and easily hurt in the social arena. I'm temperamental—the starch gave me problems emotional and mental! I'm talking bipolar (hardly stellar). The fruit and fat diet is psychologically uplifting while the starch diet is depressing, fattening and isolating: Then the thickened ectomorph tries to go along with the crowd, thinking the loud is better than the sob. They can't make it on purely fruit— the sugar excites binges and even more emotional catastrophes. What is left? Fat, protein and the daily fast: Now into a higher role she's been cast. In her own stream, the superior woman competes with no one. Now, she's a shoe-in.

GOOD EICOSANOIDS FROM FAT

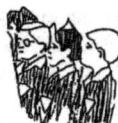

All humans are made to love fats: Modern paleo-science also shows that like a cat man needs animal fats and that's why they taste so good to him. It all comes down to the good vs. bad eicosanoids which are controlled through diet (see Just Skip Dinner). The good eicosanoids come from fat and the bad from sugar and starch. The good eicosanoids from fat are the glue holding the human body together and the most powerful agents known to man--the very definition of good health. When they're balanced the skin glows and the system hums along in perfect health. When the wrong ones are evoked the result is aging dry skin, arthritic aches and pains, blood clots, arterial constriction,

ARTS OF PALEO FASTING

asthma and heart disease. What an amazing way to recover: a fat-fasting vacation where things like rashes, asthmas and other nagging ailments disappear—just from eating the delicious fats you really want!. It reboots the system while slimming one down. Try the fat fast with the suggested recipes then reverse back to fruit for an extra snack.

ANA SYMPTOMS GONE

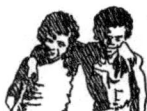

The respiratory symptoms diminish as fat elevates glucagons which opens all airways dilating all systems. What a relief as the system becomes "well-oiled" through the fat and everything opens up—and as the ugly facial swelling and discolorations dissolve. As the fat evens everything out, all excess water is released from the system! What an incredible relief! As my psychology changed I had stability and order in my food life--the desperate isolation became happy solitude combined with friendly associations. The cravings disappeared as the fat needs were met. I became a happy human being at last, a part of society and no longer called "weird". After a life of cultural indoctrination (against fat) I finally saw that society and family was nothing like I feared.

TINY BITES: BRAIN-GUT COMPETITION
Alternative to Eating Disorder Clinics

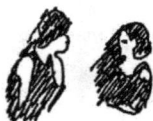

I speak to anorexics but this applies to everyone, for the benefits go across the board: Try a vacation—have a tangerine and a little guacamole or slice of cheese whenever hungry. Cheese has far more protein and fat and brings a healthy glow all day. Or just have twenty macadamia nuts spread throughout the day--now you've had your hit as a fat-fastarian-frugivore. The way you feel with mouse-meals and fasting will astound you. Now let all energy pull upward--a little while after eating you're back in the head. See how handsome/pretty properly nourished and fasting instead? Now stay there and fast all you want--as long as you include your fat or fruit you'll be fine and the wretched pecking-order systems of hospitals and controlling family hierarchies (making you want to be dead) will be over. You'll ascend to higher mental levels, be separate from sick systems and find God who designed you for a purpose. You'll have all the benefits of recovery, fasting, ladyhood and the best thing of all: freedom. I start break-fast with an early raw milkshake with yogurt/minimal fruit. Soon after maybe a chicken breast and later I think: where has all the hunger gone? This is adaptation to a new level—as the gut shrinks the brain enlarges. As a nervous fruitarian for twenty years I never would have believed I could live on so little. In my nervosa I was using gluttonous fruit-eating as a way to release emotions while staying thin. It's an entirely new fat-fruitarian-fastarian world with fatty mouse-meals then the fast to win.

WHERE HUNGER? ETERNITY IN MOUSE-MEALS

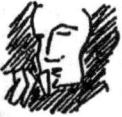

When in the eating state the energy is pulled down to the gut out of the head and you lose the consciousness of miracles. You're in dense dys-synchrony: tunnel-vision and diligence ending in frustration. In the fasting state the energy stays high in the brain and now you're clear: hello magic synchronicity as you're now totally receptive to the moment where past and future unite. It is pithy with new excitements and joys, new thoughts and fascinating avenues of discovery. You're in a much higher dimension as in an instant depression has turned to elation! Fasting has been known to heal schizophrenia and phobias instantaneously so many psychological problems may come from just our favorite foods. Allergy determines craving: we crave what we are allergic to as allergy and addictive craving are the same thing.

NO MODERN FOOD
Bad Food Ends in Jail or Out on Your Tail

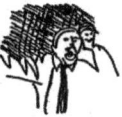

Eating modern food means we wear everything we eat, we become effete and start to cheat. Constantly elevated insulin from starch and sugar (carbohydrate other than fruit) leaves the body full of disease-storage and a suppressed immune system. This the lovely but lonely anorexic does not need. All of the modern killer diseases are due to the high-carb diet which puts us in storage mode and constricts the arteries. This tragedy is a direct result of the AMA scaring people away from fabulous fat and the protein which contains it. When the anorexic tries to stay thin on "just a little cereal" or macaroni she eventually becomes a scrawny wrinkled old crone. Don't do things that way—transcend the low-fat dogma today so the wrinkled prune (or balloon) in putting down the spoon (all afternoon after eating fat) becomes normal with high-immune.

ARTS OF PALEO FASTING

THE A.M.A. IN DIET CONFUSION

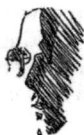

The entire A.M.A. is in confusion over diet. Despite a new vocal group of lowcarb specialists speaking out against refined carbohydrate most still tow the line regarding a low-fat diet—they are "politically correct" and increasingly going vegan. Few have the knowledge or polemical ability to fight this fat-phobia and these dry-dull diets that are evolutionarily discordant. Since the death of Atkins the low-fat voices have swooped down to invalidate his theories. Fortunately the paleo-scientists like Tom Billings have show how immuno-suppressive refined starches are: ten thousand years is not enough time for man to adapt to a new diet of refined carbs like pastas. The body yells: "what is this you're giving me?" Not knowing how to handle it, it stores it all. And thus keeping fat off the frame is a constant battle in this culture. If one craves cereals in the morning, why not substitute with raisins and nuts (pure paleo) which tastes fantastic yet immediately goes to work to sculpt the frame and eliminate residue--rather than cereals mixed with milk which only irritate and store?

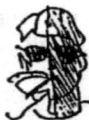

It's the med pros bringing us low—making us want to drink, use and blow. We all know the medical profession is in confusion if we think about it--for every doctor one talks to has a different opinion about a particularly diet. Many doctors just tow the current line for business or fear of disapproval--we're talking politics here. What medicine needs is a consistent paradigm: medical science must come back as a true science based on truth not politics. Many a true scientist is blackballed from university staffs because they refuse to accept the current school of thought. Since when does consensual validation determine truth? Most of the medical profession maintains low-fat is the way, the truth and the light. You now know the opposite is the case. The problem is refined sugar and starch combined with fat—animal fat alone or with fruit is the maximum health-giver.

P.S. : DRINKS

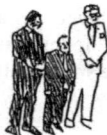

Alcohol. If you wish to drink I can't stop you. But just remember that excessive alcohol disinhibits—it dulls as it lulls you into temporary insanity. There are two ways to drink: getting drunk or enjoying leisurely wine with your meal. Choose the second: you wish to enjoy your life and feel not reel. We wish to *intensify*:

increasingly amplify our experience of the abundant environment and fast to increase fidelity to that higher experience. You're as neurotic as the petty detail you're in—stay clear, eternal and universal. Dullness from obsessive drinking drags down to details and disaster. In the old days it was seen as a "conduit to the devil" as demons come through to act through the drinker—this is the lower reptile and we all have this un-lovely tiger inside.   Instead when you feel like drinking, just fast: let your eyes go off to eternity. Drunkenness is turning the light off while fasting is turning it on.

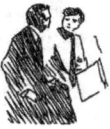

Water. The medical profession exhorts us to "drink 8 glasses of water a day". So much water drinking is unnatural and is specifically tied to the cultural diet of dry grains, refined carbohydrate and salty miscombined concoctions (salty meats without starch are ok, since glucagons eliminates water from the kidneys). When stuffed with starch or being dry from so much insulin-elevation, of course we need a lot of water! Water drinking is necessitated only by dead dry concentrated food creating acid. These foods are only ten percent water while fruit is between 80-95% water. Nuts and seeds are also only 5% water but they are paleo (we've adapted) and so   potent that only a few are needed to curb appetite and they blend perfectly with fat or high-water fruit.

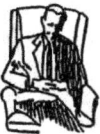

Coffee. I used to love my morning coffee but now it's acid-burn all the way. In Berg's tables coffee is a cleanser—to a rate of six, as fast as a grape! I found it delicious and exhilarating and now they've even found it is filled with more antioxidants than fruits and especially vegetables. Oh I know how the whole world—vegan or non-vegan alike—exhorts us to stop the coffee. Why? They want to eat beans, bread and rice but not coffee? I see too many contradictions in the gainsayers of this wonderful morning drink enjoyed around the world. I look so forward to my early risings with a big pot of coffee, my computer and lovely music.   If I need water I get it in my coffee and my big pitcher of lemon aid which feels so good on sun-drenched tissues in the afternoon. As Ehret said: "drink your coffee and smoke if you must—but do not eat."

REST BEFORE RULE

ARTS OF PALEO FASTING

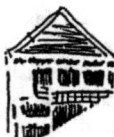

An age-old therapy for anorexics is bed rest. Why is this? Because of the hypersensitive's acute reactivity to the *constant chaos and encroachment* felt by all cerebrotonics. After a lifetime of being misunderstood, rejected and isolated--she is exhausted! The prescription for new life is: eating right, fasting while thinking of only happy holy things and getting a lot of needed rest. Anas must go through the rites of passage: fasting on people, habit and food in a long period of convalescence. Divorce from the immoral culture (sex sin, tiresome one-upping and combative message boards and all past or present rejecters) and then just read spiritual things, take walks in nature, open up to pet therapy (unconditional love), listen to lovely self-chosen music and watch great old clean movies with depth, meaning and beauty. Look out the window and thank God you made it through the horrific negative ana life phase—be glad you're not half-crazed. Now rest and look forward to the new life God has blazed, at which you'll soon be amazed!

High As A Kite Break-Fast Drink

In Blender 8 oz raw milk, cup plain (never lowfat) yogurt, 2 tab almond butter, tab coconut meat, one cube mango. WOW. Enjoy five hours totally in the now.

54

FEAST or FAST
(tunnel-vision or eternity?)

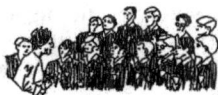

To be creative we must be happy, thin, unblocked (clean colon), undistracted, fasting most of each day--and *alone* (that's our throne)

THEIR GOD IS THEIR BELLY

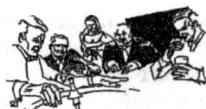

There's a black and white difference between feasting and fasting consciousness. The binger gets into TV while the faster gets into music. It's all a matter of depth: while fasting, each moment becomes pithy and fat with meaning but a tunnel-vision of irritation sets in with binging consciousness which may go on for months or years. How long? An event happens--lost love, intrusion, pessimism--and the binge starts and continues. Can an alcoholic prognosticate the duration of his drinking? No: It's just like someone in an abusive relationship who must hit bottom to get out, for that's the nature of addiction--it cannot be planned or stopped until crisis intervenes, for once started it must go through the cycle. It's up to the food-devils how long it lasts once we've taken that first binge bite.

PORN AND PAYBACK

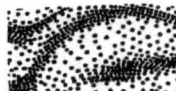

It's very frustrating for the champions where debauched thugs make millions--the gross and vulgar are applauded and rich while the genius misfit is maligned and broke. Are we really supposed to give into our basest desires while sex diseases rage? The plan I give you results in true pleasures transcending the sordid life as we enter the stream of fastarian consciousness instead. Good wholesome creativity is so much more fun and it's greatly magnified through fruit-fat-fastarianism. True genius is in good taste and based on "stern" self-discipline. This the herd hates and will even attack one for it. Why doesn't he

55

ARTS OF PALEO FASTING

want to slide down to hell with the others? Why can't he just be like the other family members? The truth is they all want to be happy, wise and thin--but lack the guts to do it the "hard" (though blissful) way. Eating wrong foods makes man passionate, violent, pugnacious and craving for more. Blockbuster movies like Troy are just violence and extended shots of the "hunk": Where is the attention to detail and the truly erotic suggestion of the subtle? The fine appreciator disdains the football huddle—the competitive strife and knife of the roman coliseum, preferring the museum to the muddle.

WILL POWER?

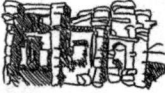

The champion is fine and refined—he's got a mind as basilic as the greatest advanced civilizations. And so he takes to fasting to increase fidelity and the same alert attention to detail. It isn't a question of will-power for the champion grows to adore fasting. The fasting consciousness is the lure for it's wonderful, pithy and four-dimensional as each moment becomes filled with miraculous insights. Life becomes multifaceted as he begins to "eat" the universe as the mind sits in the collapsed moment where past, present and future unite: this is clean, moral, pure and fun. But if one has started a binge his mind thinks of nothing but gaining satiety. The inability to gain satisfaction through an addiction compels one to keep trying and the phobia about food (a rational fear) is replaced by a magical attraction to it. Unless one eats the correct diet of fruit and fat combined with daily fasting his addiction can't be fixed, since constantly elevated insulin keeps the craving going. But there's a way to maintain the wonderful happy daily fasting life: just eat fat once a day and if still hungry later have a little fruit to clean out the residue. That fat will curtail your appetite completely. Many wish to fast each morning (enjoying this time of day the most) and then have a delicious fatty lunch. Now it's just a matter of appreciating the miraculous consciousness you'll have all afternoon. You'll begin to prefer the fast to the feast—and then see the fast as the feast. Now hold that thought for hyper-creativity that will never cease.

SYSTEMS THEORY
Hot Points of Issue

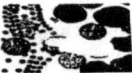

What keeps us from this state? A person can wake-up at 50 realizing he wasted his whole life seeking the attention of family members: His consciousness was eclipsed by invading elements and these became hotspots—"hot points of issue"--clouding all his thinking while blocking his higher destiny. When the others die he finally sees the insanity of it all: The sick system template assured he'd never have that attention he craved, yet the system (with him on the begging end) was etched in the brain and formed his entire identity. The day he wakes-up to the system is the happiest day of his life. Can you see the system that kept you hooked? Having finally realized the limitations of one's origins is like floating off to eternity--for it's only these hot-spots that keep us tied, tired, hungry and angry.

REJECTION IS A HOOK
And Other Lifelong Spooks

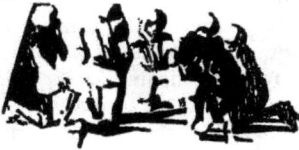

I had moved to a small cabin ten miles out of a small desert town yet for ten years I still mourned the system as if I had never left. The study of Systems theory is your therapy to get free from strife. Just see the system--was it rejection keeping you hooked? That's being spooked, for the template makes one crooked or a kook from being eclipsed by another being (that's all it took). This insight allows most victims to see how they were rooked. Being eclipsed, you're a non-entity divorced from your true self and acting out the sick system script. But now when fasting you un-hook from kooks, bad cooks and hoods on the happiest day of your life. Fasting removes the eclipse—no one is standing in your light anymore, and oh what a light-- you become a knight that very night. Gone is the blight and now we see your true beauty—what a sight and great feeling of might when free of this dragging force on consciousness (so now just fast and sit tight). The people-obstruction was a jam (of energy), a drag (on perception) and a rut (of habits to avoid anxiety). But now the sense of eternity is awe-inspiring: from bleak tunnel-vision to wide-angled vision: the prisoner is free with the power to be anything he wants, as limitless as infinity.

FASTING CONSCIOUSNESS
See The System, Gain Your Own Domain

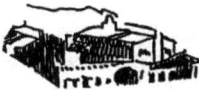

Fasting, you will see the system that kept you down. In the fast you've been with your loving God so the sick system is thrown into shocking contrast. Now let it go for it was just your war story to help others gain victory. For what keeps genius down? *Other people and the habits used to subdue the anxiety*

triggered by them, then the shame of our mal-adaptations to them. See the system, then gain your own domain—become the king of your own hacienda in the sun. Now let the fast carry you through to total world success in your field. You have a computer so with your graduate school education in systems theory—your "Ph.D. in the streets"--you have all it takes.

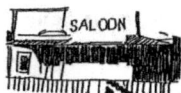

Can we say that anyone with an eating problem also has a family problem? Yes, on some level for it's the system template which has been introjected--"swallowed whole". We eat rather than love or because we can't love. The ratio of food disorders to normalcy is rising and so is the dysfunction in families. The day one finally lets a template dissolve in mind is the happiest day of his life. Oh, the relief of tension from breaking that power! I remember the day so well, when my true self swung forth into the light out of darkness and worm status. That was the day I lost respect for the eclipsing object and this has happened more than once. It is becoming mature--differentiating from human systems—after being undifferentiated (fused) with that system's collective consciousness. The other members are still fused while you're free because you refused. It is needing God not man that makes a sage or a saint after being tainted by others looking down on us. We were painted by disfavor but now whole we've got our own flavor. Enjoy it, savor and never let it go-- now from "eating disorders" we get a waiver. Our sins were hooked to the old system templates and bad memories keeping them hot. It was all a script we played out and when it dissolves, now the fun begins: diseases healed, neuroses repealed, habits yield, true or bad friendships revealed, the sinful past concealed, the curse is repealed, rising up in our field, prosperity sealed. Why? Because the template's effects were horrific and this ancient block is now removed. Herein lies happy genius, while forcing the fit to a template created only shame and remorse. Fast—on people and habits--and let those "small town blues" melt away. Fast to be the top of the heap today.

BREAK HABITS, SEE SYSTEM
Get Clear: Welcome to the Moment

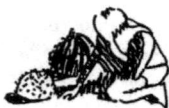

With true repentance and separation from outdated conditions and systems we open to the magnificent moment in full cornucopic detail. If one can't "see" the system set-up, then break free the other way: by refusing to give into the habit used to avoid anxiety from the template. Can you do that--refuse to give in just one time? Your life will implode open to heavenly dimensions and you'll be so happy in the morning with true pleasures forevermore. For it was that very system template that damaged vision of the whole--that fantastic perception that is *won*. Are you ready to achieve true reality today? Fast in the morning and enjoy each day as you sit in eternity— where past and future sit in the present moment. The biggest habit we must break is crudity from being part of the world. Sinful celebrities in the spotlight are compelled to bring themselves down because money and family won't instill maturity which a good publicist intends to portray, by controlling the things they say. Rather than immersion in the magic moment they're attending to the wrong details, display immaturity then get mad at their poor reviews. As they get sore, the critics pile it on some more! But if their reality shows make us snore, has not their self-esteem gone out the door way back before?

☐TO THE GREAT-GOING-DOWN
Retreat, Retrench, Repent

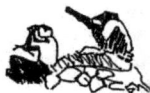

To the great-going-down: I recommend you stop all appearances, fast and pray, show gratitude that it wasn't worse than it was and then become as humble as a child. This means to retreat, retrench, and repent. Return to the elements: just you and the stars. Then, come back fresh, like Einstein: saintly, sober and mild. Stay in the loop, you'll stay riled. After sweet solitude you'll return newly self-styled (no more in reaction—that's just the ego going wild). Reality shows are the ego thinking we want to view their boring empty lives. It's the essence of idolatry, for people worshippers have no life--society's wife in reaction to strife. Great artists take years and decades to produce a perfect masterpiece (to present to a dying world who will be edified for all that work)–but never before patiently making sure it's all perfect (truly done). Slow and steady, wait until ready, then you've won. No photos unless perfect with discretion, not showing imperfection.

IN "SITU" AND CREATIVE ACTION

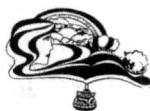

Fasting (on people, food and habits) we get more into life and we're not as hooked to the computer. We're in our own *situ*— situation: the fat moment-- and once there we may never want to stray again. We have our permanent ever-new multivariate home: the fasting consciousness. When I became a daily faster I became a desert-walker over 230 acres of wilderness for most of the day. I viewed it as a phantasmagoria while the ordinary eater sees the desert as downright desolate. It's a miracle how creativity and true perception erupts the minute bad associations and habits are released: dissolve obstruction to obtain the spiritual skies. Now, there is now no limit on your potential--you become co-creators with God and it's like a new toy.

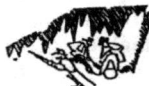

In the fat moment the holy sage is busy all day putting things into place and that is "creativity". He is re-assembling a pre-existing matrix and it's his life's work to figure it all out. What a relief that fasting alone compels completion. We've finally done it: transcended all useless burdens holding us down to this boring mundane plane, just by starting or intending to fast. This age-old spiritual method has now illuminated the path to completion, what we always wanted but remained just outside our grasp. I was happy to see my destiny was to walk in the desert, get inspired and come in to write. How simple! But in the eating consciousness this correct routine is missed—we tenaciously hold on to useless complexity thinking we're doing something great while remaining third-rate. The eater "falls into his bag"--his ruts of recycled energy in outworn or evil channels. We must find the simple unique design for each moment (for it's divine) and fasting is the fastest way to do this.

HOW CAN I FAST IF I'M A BINGER?

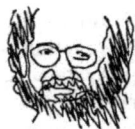

This is a constant question and I have the solution. If you're a binger continue to binge. Yes, I say binge. Binge daily at the same time but don't eat one thing at the other times. Gradually you get used to 22 hours of fasting a day without giving up your beloved precious party. When you binge don't feel guilt but think instead: "I'm doing personal research to see how (bad, sick, bloated, ugly) I feel with these foods and this necessary research will keep me from them for life." Then you begin to see how much more you enjoy the fasting times and soon you'll be able to replace very good healthy food that quells appetite for days at a time, rather than your useless empty binge food. With this change you suddenly realize how much better you feel with a little fruit or fauna--streamlining rather than protruding the mid-region. Then presto: you're a mini-faster: eating once daily of the most healthy foods. Now wasn't that simple? Don't say "can't" or "never". Just gradually move into it beginning by having your "delicious feast" once a day— without guilt, for it's your Rx. Luncheon or afternoon supper would be best, then do the opposite thing the rest of the day: fast and rest.

ARTS OF PALEO FASTING

INSULTS: OP-TRUTH
Whatever They Say, Take the Opposite View

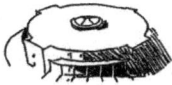

Many young women are crippled with low self-esteem from years of toxic relationships resulting in a "thin skin". Insults or even supposed rebuffs are devastating but I have a solution for that too: whatever "they" say, take the opposite view. If they call you "corny" think: "I'm the Queen: cosmic, cute, the cat's meow." Remember the slogan: "op-truth". The devil's a liar--insults indicate the culprit's at the lower level to which the Queen will not sink (that's how she stays in the pink). Instead she says "op-truth"--the opposite is true, so she keeps her cosmic view. There's another insight about insults: they always precede greater success if you deal with them right, but if you relapse in reaction you've missed the golden ring again (out goes the light). To the Queen this is sin--you must pass the test: stand strong, ignore the throng. They're all wrong but for you it won't be long. Success is sure--it's your song, so carry on. The fast is where you belong so come along: imperviously on top (and not from wearing a thong).

GETTING SKINNY
Water Retention and Cellulite

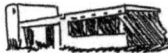

Once having rejected the "voices" from the mediocre, thorny and low-grade past, the new fastarian can't wait to dissolve fat and become thin. It may help him to know that what he sees as "fat" is mostly water retention from eating the wrong foods. Making the switch to fat elevates glucagons which instantly releases all water from the kidneys. Yes in one miraculous moment the body reverses into water-release mode, for it's part of ketosis--fat burning--to dispel water pressing on fat cells causing the appearance of cellulite. Stick to fat, fruit and fasting and all cellulite breaks up with gentle exercise such as yoga and walking: now your talking (they'll be gawking).

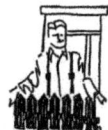

That ugly cellulite along with the "false body" is a mass of inferior (illogical) cells built by inferior foods. Stop eating anything but fruit and fat and get yourself some good walking shoes. Now shake those legs. As you take in the mountain vistas, the seas, the beautiful sky and cloud formations, the nitrogen, the gentle breeze, the crescent moon and the fabulous sunshine then walk fast and shake your legs until everything tightens up and all energy frees. When you're finally free of the lazy, immature and isolated binging life you'll be saying good-bye to the blues and blubber too.

ECTOS-FREE
Transcending People and Rejection

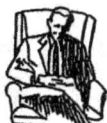

The ectomorph-cerebetonic is thin and private: This is the way he must be to be free. In his early life he lived with the Bigs and was compelled to adapt to them--and the resulting mal-adaptation was the foundation of his problems. This tension and trauma is resolved by understanding the system-matrix in which he is caught: the ecto-cereb is a hypersensitive who is most hurt by the leveling process of the herd. Because of his body-type and temperament he is least able to adapt to the big and brusque. It's a sad plight: unable to adapt yet having to, trying to stay on top while also keeping Mr. Big happy and harmless. It's essentially a war between two separate realities: left and right, outer vs. inner, cultural vs. natural, group vs. individual, West vs. East, worldly vs. spiritual, gross vs. refined. The tiny cerebetonic who finally bridges the gap becomes Top Dog—a rarity, for most die in the spirit. Good times are coming—let me tell you by summing: the ecto tends to be trivialized and minimized in the mesomorphic world: we've been slammed, called scum and scammed so today I say fast and pray then no more cry—see the sky? That's our high.

MUST HAVE PENACHE

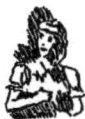

Christ was despised and rejected by man: he was "esteemed not." The Great are sided against in tribe-ulative life—a playground where the bullies persecute the small (the seemingly weak). The world says "big is more" while Truth says *less* is more. Einstein showed that most creative energy comes in least mass so the ectomorph must build character to prove this out. The best and quickest way is the fast and thus the fast is this way to true freedom. It's a war but the fasting ectomorph lets out a roar as he fights some more. When he finally gets to shore he never again stores fat or the truth—he must let it out and cut to the core. He wins the good fight and it becomes his lore (the story of his war). This is the spirit of panache: a "tuft of feathers" on the helmet: the fight is for the integrity of the true self which must prevail being designed by God for a purpose. The ectomorph survives by becoming godly or he comes off oddly.

SHAKE OFF THE HURTS:
Judgment and Disapproval

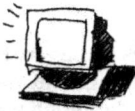

The journey of genius can be treacherous and dangerous. There's a price to pay with a strong anointing on your life—talents bring a curse, then the purse. The world can be cruel but on the internet we'll rule. Most unhappy people come from sick systems where genius is misunderstood and rejected. Fast and this won't last for it's all in the past--now who goes last? Your future is vast: into your destiny you've been cast while your history is passed—what a contrast when no more harassed.

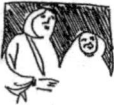

The ecto must say "I cannot adapt to them, they must adapt to me—my inaccessibility." Now you'll see how inspired you can be. Don't let the past ruin your destiny: "Rest in Me." Then you'll see how great you're meant to be. Be the King—lock them out for the more they contradict or correct your words and bring up your past the more you stay down. Ask God to heal you and quit bleeding once healed. We can survive rejection if we can learn to "shake it off" like a harmless snake or bug. Letting someone disclaim your words or your past is a mental tyranny through thought-strangulation. To the verbally vicious you must use the slogan "attack those unhappy memories." Stay high in the present moment--who you are today--for they're all made of clay: having made you their prey they're all going gray. They betray, then decay—that's mankind from the beginning so don't delay and fast to escape this cliché.

BAD FAITH OR FULLNESS

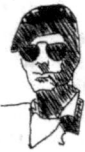

Know your enemy. Do you even know who he/she is? He may be your most trusted friend, as bad faith abounds. You may even feel a need for a useless person bringing you down. In whom do you put your faith? Once you come alert to the enemy, you're clear--as the universe alights you've no more to fear for being a seer you can perfectly steer. Without bad faith God is near so this can be your glory year (no more tears). To the Daily Fast you must adhere: by going austere your reward is near so make it your career then open new frontiers and enjoy your premier--for you'll be a star once the bad disappears. You'll need a financier but only if those friends can't interfere. To be a successful pioneer, *simply persevere.*

NOW IS THE TIME
Too "Weird" to Live, Too Rare to Die

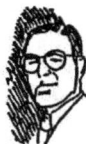

Now is the time for all good men to come to the for--out of the obscure periphery being controlled by inferiors. Do you feel misjudged, maligned or identity-murdered? You're in a sick system keeping you down. The superior man must rise up for he cannot be controlled by people and God Almighty too. The time has come to lose your numb and don't be so dumb. You're a plum being thrown a crumb! Just think what you can become not being treated like scum. The trick is to not succumb when seen as a bum: avoid the rum and you won't end in slum. For just look where you've come from (you've grown much more than some). Now just continue to hum along in your own stream beating your drum. You've got me for a chum for I know what it's like being stuck in black gum even while having a green thumb. The future holds a grand sum but only if you stay away from.

3 OBSTRUCTIONS: PEOPLE, HABIT, FOOD

Dissolving obstruction on any level brings changes on all other levels: Because of the interaction between debris (food), memory (templates and habits) and people (culture, family, associates) one can dissolve templates by breaking other parts of the chain: Sudden dissociation from evil elements shocks the body-brain into transformation—psychic opening or aperture syndrome. A long fast can force this break so that habits and templates dissolve--but a diligent daily fast can do the same. Repentance from bad habits dissolves templates determining associations while vanquishing old food cravings. People, habits or debris are the three obstructions: work on one, transform the others as well. You're about to break through your shell (even though you fell).

BREAK YOUR TEMPLATES OR DIE
Cultural Neurosis: Splits are the Pits

ARTS OF PALEO FASTING

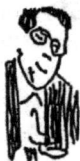

The "herd" sees everything alike. For most neurotic templates are confirmed by culture: There's a continuous feedback between the sick system and the culture of stereotypic "splits": old vs. young, male vs. female, rich vs. poor. This cultural neurosis is present in all cultures to a degree: everyone feels diminished at some point when confronted with these put-downs. To these projections the isolate says "NO": having released culture he's the True Self, ever-superior and never slighted. Devices of the sick system are magnifications of culturally-confirmed values like sexism or ageism and all cultures are "sick" in different degrees: *the more dense the more split and conformist.* In seeking outside help an abused female is likely to face the same stereotypes in society as she does in her own home so what can she do but settle for less? And then you have the ana-ectomorph who must be free to see and to be. As a system-refugee in great relief she becomes a reclusee: the Queen Bee. If she can ever find a man who can appreciate these differences she'll be filled with glee, for in a good tree ectos is made more free--the healthy system maintains the Renaissance Man/Woman as true genius is increasingly released through spiritual awakening: the contagion of enlightenment (and it's all for free).

WATCH WHAT YOU PUT IN YOUR FACE

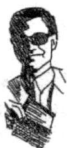

How the theory is high-tech: Cultural conformity and family dysfunction is correlated with eating styles. Bad eating hardens the body into a statue of fixed action patterns that never seem to change: gabbing and gorging. The result: all doors closed to further opportunity. Watch what (and who) you put in your face, for it will leave a trace. You must have space from the maize of people, habits and food for it's these flesh and world obstructions that make you rude. An eating disorder creates mental chaos and then disfavor as one is pooh-poohed. Destiny is blocked by the food for which you lusted, God's plans that you busted or the people you trusted.

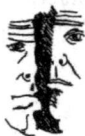

Starch makes one lopsided and split. Ehret said that alcohol, meat and coffee are relatively harmless compared to the common starchy concoctions. The problem is non-paleo food: anything other than plants, nuts and fauna. Daily fast so the immune system is set free to defend against the rest—that is best. The food we need—fruit or fat—requires very little by the elite. In my estimation vegetables will make you effete (see "veggies are for rabbits"). Never eat at frustration, for contrary to public opinion eating always makes things worse. If you fast

ARTS OF PALEO FASTING

(not feast) at disappointment consciousness will pop (open) and lock (no more relapse) into a brand new dimension bringing solutions to all problems: It's the *frustration of the fires of desire* that brings this release. This generation hates all authority—even self-made rules like fasting plans--as the minute craving starts out goes the plan. By understanding the psychodynamics of frustration and then "hurting to go higher" just one time creates such joy we long to follow our own rules—and those who can't become fools. Fast: face the fires of desire, deny frustration, receive reward.

AVOID THE DILATORY

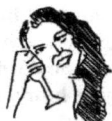

What an incredible waste of time waiting for people. Wouldn't it be better just to fast and wait on God? Never set appointments with those who come late or not at all. This is self-esteem: Here we're the Queen but they've become mean as they break our routine. Stay with those who respect your time--then life becomes sublime (serene).   Once rid of those acting thirteen you can easily become lean and you'll have the sheen. Guard your time. I'll say it in rhyme: keeping you waiting means they're third-rating you (that's when genius gets blue). Why maintain this shoddy crew—you mean you want their approval too? Herein lies the basis of food disorder and addiction: If I want all to like me they would so rule and control my life I'd fall from destiny. If your priority is social approval your genius will take you to shame not fame— the "bad act." Just pursue your own talent with a bag over your head. Stay free: never look 'em in the eye just look up to your rich Daddy in the sky.

WIN AT SOCIOLOGY: BE GOD'S PRODIGY

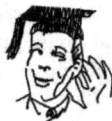

Few friends at the end. We all have "slips" but these relapses disclose who our friends are, resulting in the drastic pruning and chopping process just preceding success. The humiliation of having sunk to a lower previous level brings the decision to cast the entire level out—bad habits and the associates maintaining them— to become greater than before the sin cycle began. I pray you survive your pre-success crises for the bounty will be unbelievable if you do.

Be humble, meek and sweet. Let me give you a tip: watch your lip. You may want to rip right into those who oppose you, the rose. I suppose as one who knows genius always has lows. I say go solo or you'll go so-low as they blow

ARTS OF PALEO FASTING

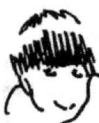

you down like ducks in a row. So never tow their line for you gotta get spine—that means shine. Now draw your line: win at sociology—be God's prodigy. That's tautology, not pomposity but a grand life-eulogy. While gaining your freedom, poise and patience are necessary to sever the attachment to lower elements without relapsing back into them.

INDEPENDENCE DAY

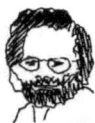

Become independent—transcend the social world which is either constantly shifting alliances or the other extreme: rigid scapegoat systems that never change. Attempts to adapt bring insanity in the cerebrotonic for whom the only answer is to fast and elevate above the cobweb-illusions of human interactions. Look down on the herd as you fly above like a bird. Cosmic man is able to muse at the folly of human interaction, having seen the system that kept him down--for if he stays stuck he's getting the rug pulled out continuously and that the superior man cannot stand. Go within--that's your twin. Now you can stay thin. Take all else on the chin, wear a grin. You may have to avoid your kin (it's no sin) for where they're concerned you've got a thin skin to your chagrin. Fast, for the time has come to begin.

SOCIAL ADDICTION AND HYPNOTISM

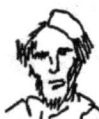

Social addiction and hypnotism are synonymous. Out of low self-esteem one seeks social back-pats and if he can't he falls into depression. Even those who are benefited by the social scene fear rebuffs. But alone in nature, man clears: Suddenly (despite far less distractions) he's never bored, lonely or depressed. Like any other addiction social hypnotism is: needing it more but enjoying it less. Have no contact with evil. Sign nothing, stop what you're doing and fast. Let God Almighty work for you as you hide in His wings. It's like a well of living water coming up like springs. So many blessings from the richest diet of Kings! When free of fakers you'll see them as empty, so fast for vision (so it's just the truth that rings).

BLESSINGS HIGHER THAN CURSINGS

68

ARTS OF PALEO FASTING

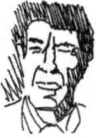

The spiritually mature make mistakes but they know what to do about it: Just repent and go on. Sullen self-shame is childish. Don't worry over your rep with people, always trying to placate or please. The people-pleaser eventually learns that people will only manipulate and control, then dump when done. The social whirl makes your values curl--you're no call-girl so end this thankless swirl. Find instead the pearl of great price: Just please God--let Him give you a good rep. It'll be far higher and more permanent than what's achieved with man, who has a short attention span. He care's only for his clan so you'll always feel less than. So here's the new game plan: Fast— you can. The godless group is like the Klan (always feeling better than) but the Fast has been the way out since time began. The social reality is a flash but a fake. It overtakes the mind until it's all you can take. Come home to your own stream where there is no competition: that's a cake-walk. You've been caught in a painful syndrome but now your life shines like chrome: it's like a beautiful dome (ohm). Find your own niche, never again to roam.

WE'VE BEEN IN FOG BUT NOW THEY'LL RESIGN

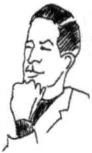

Think about it: We've been in a fog due to blind faith in treacherous people. They were popular with idiots and we were not, so we saw them as superior (their approval we sought). We were guilty of idolatry (people-worship, even the rot). But now with the faster's vision we want their removal (freedom from disapproval). Now we know the foe, we seek the divine: the ones who are fine. Through the fast we have the shine—a shrine and a sign of spine. Transcend the swine and their constant whine. This life of mine is what's on the tree and vine (watch the wine) and the fast to assign. I know how to combine lest destiny decline (that's my life in the Grand Design). If they continue to malign they'll have to resign, for me and my associates must be kind.

DEEP AS SEAS FOODS LIKE THESE

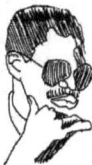

The way to world peace is the riddance of blood-irritants like refined starch. To separate from white mush makes one very high as all energy elevates to the head and shoots through every cell. The nitrogen (air) and solar radiation (sun) is our highest nutrition as the body re-adapts to getting it all from these invisible but far richer sources. In the brain the figure inverts with

ARTS OF PALEO FASTING

the ground as everything is seen in reverse: We go from fear of deprivation to complete faith in glorious miracles for our benefit. Eat fat and fruit then fast— you've come home at last while all problems are resolved (they're all in the past).

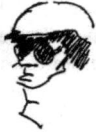

When a soldier lay down his arms he's at the mercy of his captors. If you can't defend yourself they can shoot you and no one cares. Your only defense is God, fasting and the correct fuel for Man the fauna-frugivore. So give up the vice: it's not nice all that rice. Just have a slice: of fruit or fat (these are the keys). You'll be as deep as the seas made by foods like these. As a famous leader once said "if you want peace you must prepare for war." The fasting champ is ready for problems every moment—he never gets complacent--but his weapons are spiritual: eating (as God designed) and fasting is his destiny as it makes even the foe admire his courage and sincerity.

DAILY FASTING IS A RARE ACHIEVEMENT

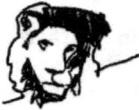

It's the fact that you fast daily that both indicates and makes you Great. Your highness is the unique me-ness, no more a mess while they could care less. Daily fasting is an achievement of a very few while everyone else seems blue. It's a matter of staying paleo-true so the protein-nourished spirit can come through. To the cultural crass and raw vegan sass we bid adieu—it's a matter of who's who, for the future's ours and in full view: all things new, prosperity to accrue. Now let your mind renew and save the past just for review—what a shampoo! You've repented, so guilt and shame are taboo. The fast divides you from the past as your dreams can now ensue and your genius comes through. You'll be saying to God "thank you" as all your wishes come true.

MAN THE EMBODIED EXPERIENCER
Memory Stored in the Body

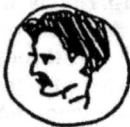

The body is who we are. Experience originates in the body beneath the neck. This is memory—holographically stored in tissue. Man reacts to situations not from his frontal cortex (reasoning) but rather from his automatic body holograms (stored in the muscles and GSR—galvanic skin response). An example is "colon science." Months of enemas rid the victim

70

of the terrible depression locked in fecal matter, a very low vibration determining attitude and memory. The fast dissolves all layers of memory— the "stuff" of depression. It's elating to go forward—to dis-entrench from past mistakes and all systems keeping you down. You'll be amazed at how dissolving the body-mind by frustrating desire deletes the past. Bad memories are gassed, our foes are outclassed, and the future is vast. Looking back when you were an outcast makes you aghast, for what a contrast! Never forget it was all due to obstruction—that's why you were harassed, but now you're unsurpassed.

CHANGE ROUTINES: REVERSE DIETS

I myself prefer monotony but you may prefer changing your routines—some days just distilled water with some lemon, some days just mono-fruit and some days breakfast-only with doughless pizza, fish or chicken followed by a fast to next a.m. break-fast, the next day or for the entire week-end. You learn to read your needs and that's the variety here: not of tastes but of speeds (cleansing or rebuilding actions). Each change creates a different reality—the spice of your new life. Though it seems austere these changes bring exciting variety of joy. It's your new toy keeping you poised so trifles won't annoy while your fat is destroyed.

EAT THEN ATTRACT, RE-INVENT

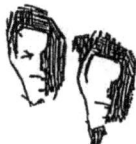

Our slogan "eat then fast" could also mean "eat, fast then *attract*." Think of all the benefits from fasting rather than the deprivation of "eating." Begin to see eating as losing and fasting as winning—all ideas, contracts, health, wealth. You can now re-invent yourself with any new problem. You'll have the clarity to go to higher archetypes—then it's your choice which fairytale you play. There is power in archetypes so you'll be instantly re-pegged in the herd mind. Always be kind and gentle, for the fast is the fastest way to re-identity yourself and this will mean witty inventions to the highest degree. It's more than that—it's the very key from which all-bad will flee. It's a joyous spree, a new family-tree where all will agree. When rid of debris God puts out a new decree: "make this one a Grand Marquis." You'll be satisfied like me (for whom it's a constant jubilee).

The END--completion--will take care of itself. There's an inertia towards completion/no more insults.

ARTS OF PALEO FASTING

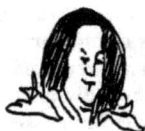

In humid weather the body gets dumpy. It seems to expand while the spirit becomes turgid, slow, laborious. But fasting breaks this cord: you won't be bored as your spirit comes from the Lord. Fast, elongate—then it's a new trait as you attract a mate (it's never too late). You're now first-rate so you'll win out the gate. You won't have to fight your enemies--by your rejection you've already won. Because you've chosen the higher way, destiny takes over on your side. Nothing to do, no one to see—just fast and enjoy the ride. You must know you've won and that Victory is sure and soon (if it's only in the Lord you confide).

BURNING BUILDING SYNDROME
Dealing with the Trauma of Flip-Flops

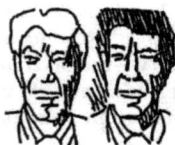

How to deal with hostile environments and vacillations. It's bad not having control in your own situation. That's the anorexic—feeling weak and dominated in the land of the bigs and the brusque. She feels trapped in this syndrome: a "burning building" without escape--except when fasting which puts her on "top" of impossible situations. They say of the faster: "pictures don't do her justice—it's her aura which glows." It's a question of flesh vs. spirit: to deny the flesh the spirit takes over instead and it shows how to be led. For example, a perfect (reconstructed) intestine and stomach is in the ethereal body (a template-seed) which, in a high-energy body occurs quickly with fruit and fasting. The fruit itself is a natural wonder by the effect it has on the body and the fast is even quicker—both are God's marvels, especially when combined with the ray. Just feel your, trunk, legs and arms elongate in the sun! To be a body mystic you must love your body for good, for the dense are unrelated to their body except to use it for hedonistic purposes—otherwise it's like wood.

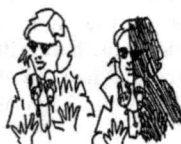

As you distinguish yourself from the masses of asses you will be relieved to know the mesomorphs have no memories of you except that you were "trivial". It is only food and toxins that tie us into eating society—release, and release! Love nature as your fasting body clarifies, not so much "natural foods" but the supernatural processes of the fasting body—no food! As the intestine reconstructs itself so does the face and the lung. Now you're becoming "silky" and "lustrous" looking. It's higher, wiser, richer as we fearlessly fly to higher places as God gives us all things to

72

ARTS OF PALEO FASTING

enjoy divinely—this is eternity! Let the fast and pure God-given talent take you to the top. If you're a daily faster you'll win till you drop and never be a flop. So don't stop--avoid that pizza shop or just eat the top.

☐TRIBULATION IS EVERYWHERE
Fear Not Evil

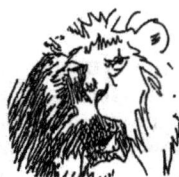

Tribulation is everywhere, but fear not evil. Just say "I don't want to argue. My creative ideas are my own." Come in from the cold, to enjoy total inner protection. Regard the outer as a theatre with you as audience--mere practice for you as their leader (later). That's the dance, the fast is your lance and the last chance. Now with fruit and the fat we're living in France: It's a wonderful stance as your new energy makes you jump and prance (attracting more than a glance). This trip is a trance, it's an advance to self-enhance and good for finance. So now just view the expanse: this is romance! Do a sun dance by no more tolerating their song-and-dance. Right action brings right fruit and wrong action brings wrong fruit. One right action is to avoid all peace-stealers--like fruitless arguing, anger or waiting for those who love keeping you waiting. Remember, when God wants to help you he sends a person, and when the devil wants to destroy you he sends a person! You must fast to discern: learn or burn, spurn then earn.

STAY AUSTERE—YOUR REWARD IS NEAR

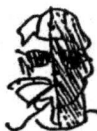

Know your enemy, and watch who you put your faith in. You may be shocked to see it's your "trusted friends" of years driving you to tears. In your mal-adaptation to false friends you've become dull and blunted (denial takes a toll on perception) and life has been grating, not humming: by your mere association you've been kept in the rears. Once you become alert and fastgloriously clear you're now free of faker-fears. A clean slate precedes greatest success: For greatest accomplishments affecting the whole world you must keep starting over again, resuming only with trusted (proven, not rusted) people around. If you can do that success is sure, but if not you'll remain confound. Now starts the good cheer if you give me an ear on how to proceed in highest gear: Don't make decisions if it's not in your vision—if you don't feel peace about something regarding your career. Just stay home and fast so God is near: let Him be your whole sphere. If you can relax into faith this is your glory year, if to the daily fast you adhere: Stay austere and your reward is near. Make fasting your career pursuant to new frontiers, then get ready for your premier. You'll be a bright star once that bad influence disappears, and you'll even need a financier if you stop letting those "friends" interfere. To be a successful pioneer all you need is to follow this plan, then persevere.

MAN IS OLIGIPHAGOUS

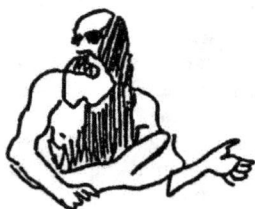

The less variety in your diet the more efficient in overcoming obstructions. Superior species are *oligiphagous*: this means maximally existing on fewest varieties, and you'll have only two: fruit or fat. Low-variety equals optimal adaptation: if you eat only two categories of paleo foods your body quickly adapts beautifully, maximizing this superior blend. This concept is the opposite to common diet dogma of eating multi-varieties to "ensure getting all the vitamins". The body reconstitutes anything we eat to maximize our needs. Fruit or fat (my preference) once a day can be a permanent diet with perfect elimination. It's actually continuous fasting punctuated by the perfect frugal foods for man, the fauna-frugivorous-fastarian. Forget eating everything on earth (it's all for the other animals too).

LIFE A CONTINUOUS FAST

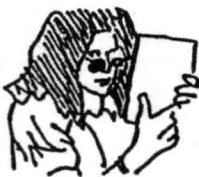

Once you've taken your daily dosage of fruit and fat there's no reason to eat again. We eat from boredom or stomach inflammation (cleansing) which we mistakenly call "hunger pain". Cut back. If you feel sick, go to bed until it passes for you're fasting for a successful future--a good-looking centenarian so slick after the gut-encumbrance out-kicks. Never eat at boredom and eat only to keep from starving. Eat raisons to bind up the mucus causing the pain. Keep juggling your diet according to your current needs. Are you suffering today? Time to do something different--reverse gears into more fruit, fasting or fat and less or none of what you've been doing. If you're fighting a craving why not persevere and become a soldier of self? Soon as your body adapts to the new routine these symptoms will disappear so look

ARTS OF PALEO FASTING

ahead to be the magic elf. Soon you'll have made gold with your new life free of cravings--and old jealousies and resentments at their base will be gone instead. Forget what you dread (what they said) and just look ahead. Drink distilled water tinged with lemon because much "hunger" is actually thirst. Fast for a budget cut as you shrink that gut. Make it tiny as a walnut and see it as a rut for the eating life you must cut—they'll all watch as you strut.

NO AB MACHINES
☐GUARDING WHAT GETS IN

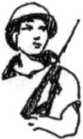

The ectomorph is an hyperevoloute-neanthrope highest on the evolutionary ladder. This is the New Man, the Superior Man, the Renaissance Man. He is on a proprioceptive journey from which there is no return. To maximize the trip he must be hypervigilant: he must guard what gets in his body, environment and mind. Due to his hypersensitivity he must have high boundaries—the highest of anyone—lest he become the worst of the lot. Before he becomes exclusive, he cries a lot because of all the inappropriate rot he bought but when he learns to just do his work he wins the whole pot. Always wear a hardhat: influence them but don't let them influence you. Be vigilant: watch for miracles like a cat watches a mouse hole, and watch what gets in!

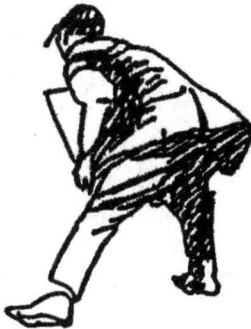

Fast and you'll need no ab-machine for all those ugly rolls and cellulite will automatically tighten up and go away. Exercise may help but nothing de-ages and repairs like the fast: On a scale the fast is a ten, exercise is a one. If you can fast after breakfast why postpone it until after lunch? It's the fasting consciousness that gives you the hunch! With great expectation of this wonderful routine you won't postpone it again, for digestion brings quirks but fasting brings world success in all your works. It's being God's bride, much more exciting than a life like Bonny and Clyde. You'll start to glide with heaven as your guide. The fast will save your hide so fast with pride (even after fried). Now you're entering the great divide—as you fast you'll go worldwide and be oversupplied: Carnivores eat fruit and leaves. It's a matter of proportion, which varies.

DEPRESSION
Deep Darkness Could Be a Wake-Up Call

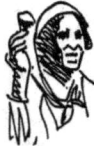

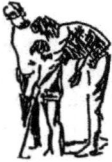

As a young child I was always into projects and lessons and thrived on a paleo diet that most mothers prepared in the fifties. Later as a fruitarian—after an initial "high"--I sank into darkness and got so low I wanted to blow this place without a trace. Depression is a worldwide epidemic and a terrible thing to experience—uselessness, hopelessness, lost fascination, bore-dumb. I never want to experience it again. With this reversal dieting plan every day is happy and humming but before this I spent half my time in "fruitless" bipolar extremes and many downs. Finally the True Self called out for fauna: animal protein and fat. I took my fauna meals at a swank restaurant surrounded by beauty and bounty and bounced back instantly. From that food-switch I went from begging for mercy to bragging on God. Eat fauna when down--your immunity's enhanced and your mind's entranced. The low-fat (fat-phobic) culture is rampant with depression but when properly fed the fastarian brain breaks out and shoots up. Once properly fed, think on these things:

HEARTBREAK IN THIS WORLD

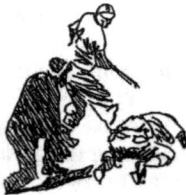

Is that ache in the gut from a people rut or something you chose (refused to cut)? To escape this painful darkness it's the world (your "friends") and the past we must close. Don't worry over changes—just ride with what God arranges. We gain strength from what lies behind, but still the present reality must be redefined. It is sad when we wakeup from being blind but seeing ourselves and others brings out the royal qualities of patience making us kind. It doesn't help to be wined and dined for afterwards it's back to the same old

76

ARTS OF PALEO FASTING

grind unless God enters the mind. People can be so cruel--but if you'll fast and look upward (blend your life and His as one) this depression you can shun. Trust him with changes lest the mind deranges. For all your tears He sees and your reward is soon (you'll be greatly pleased). Make a list of all you need, and see how dependency on false friends made you weak-kneed. God will give you help from other directions and you're be freed.

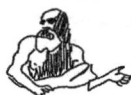

If it's with this earthly life you've signed you can easily lose your mind for it's over in a minute--only trusting God gives you shine. How to leave depression behind: Focus on God *for it's you He designed*. Happily living just this fasting day is more exciting than all else combined. So leave past and future to Him for all else is too unkind. Focusing on this world is like flying blind for it's a sleazy lot, mankind—we've been maligned as our genius was declined. But fast and you'll leave the doldrums behind for you've been redefined if with God you're aligned.

NO MORE UNDERMINED
Be a Catcher of the Lecher and Soul-Snatcher

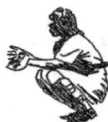

Catch all bad thoughts and influences and delete to the trash. You've no need to be redesigned, just no longer undermined. Through labels like "old", "fat" or "dumb" we've been confined but through God and angels our genius is enshrined. It's with God's angelic gang you're now intertwined, so just relax and do your work and only of God and his nurturing angels should your heart remind. Keeping your mind on these things will produce perfect peace, then your joy won't cease. With your mind stayed on Him, things below go strangely dim. Think of the angels as your kin. The world's caprice will all decrease if on your mind you use this thought-police: all thoughts of world, man, past and future you must now release. Now it's a snap to fast and your joy will increase as you're no more obese. Do what I did: go to a fancy restaurant with beautiful surroundings and have your cheese omelet or fish dish. See yourself as a major VIP as you take in the majestic ambience and think of the glory that lies ahead. Eat your fill then get ready with great expectancy of the miracle you're about to see. Spend all day fasting in reverie and wild imaginings of the best that you can be at the top of the family tree. No matter what you're at the apex of life, a magic jubilee if you fast all day with your mind on God (and it's all for free).

ARTS OF PALEO FASTING

HUMAN TIDE OR GOD'S BRIDE?

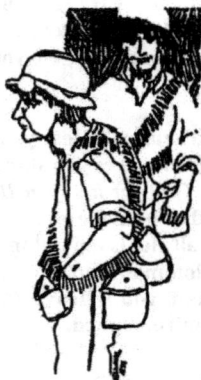

The world's gone mad and bad. But draw near to God and He'll draw near to you. Humbly repent and he'll lift you up. As newly righteous you'll not be moved if you put no confidence in man but all in God. Trust not in friends nor guide. Only in God—be His bride while from all those chumps you hide. Go higher now: it's a matter of self-esteem and pride—for that masochist trip is not your ride (you must prevent the downward slide). With only God it's constant joy as blessings flow so just ride the tide! As for man, take him in stride: Insults and social rebuffs--leave it all aside for it's a constant collide (especially in those you did confide). So decide: let them continue to deride or from them divide then go inside. God will provide if you and Him coincide (then your work and fame can spread worldwide).Yes world and man is a can of worms. Man the worm is flimsy (infirm). He vacillates, he's vile, he contaminates like germs. If you're spiritual and smart he's compelled to make you squirm. Come to terms: only God confirms. Know this score for depression no more. Transcend the world then God cleans to the core to make you strong, so let out a roar! Fasting is the answer to all your problems galore.

DIVINE DESTRUCTION OF DEEP DARKNESS

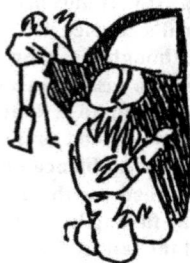

Just do your work and avoid the smirk. Thank God for past blessings--this builds trust that your current problems will also be solved. Only think on good things (staying happy) never bad things (staying sad). As you think in your heart so are you. Delight yourself in God and He shall give you the desires of your heart. Commit your way and then rest in Him—wait patiently for Him. "They that wait on the Lord shall renew their strength." Whenever you feel sorrow take it to God. "They cried to the Lord in their trouble and He saved them from ALL distresses." "If you abide in Me ask what you will and it shall be done for you." But live defensively: expecting the promised tribulation in life means you won't be surprised when it comes. "We must through tribulation enter the Kingdom of God. Many are the afflictions of the righteous but the Lord delivers them from them all." "We are troubled on every side yet not distressed. Our light affliction is but for a moment yet works a far exceeding and eternal weight of glory'. Set your mind on things above so things below go "strangely dim". Seeking God first means all things are added unto you. Don't borrow problems from yesterday or tomorrow (enough problems just today). You'll forget all your misery if you just live this moment and the elements—enjoy the wind and ray.

THE KEY TO SUCCESS

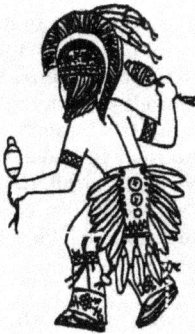

The key to success is remembering who gives it to you: God! Don't let arrogance and pride take over or you'll again sink in your own swill (you will). It's harder to deal with sudden fame and money than it is to deal with sin and tragedy. You must stay humble and always thank God, then your success will be lasting. No matter what stay mild and meek like a child—don't change because the world is (with you) beguiled. If you stay meek you'll maintain maximum favor with God and man and rise to your peak. Don't chance "first fame syndrome"—called "first" because the overnight success is followed by a sudden fall from grace and disappearance. Then there's a long period of building back up to true success (if it ever happens again). The problem is that as the years pass it's much harder—our sins aren't "cute" anymore and the creative well runs dry (we become a bore). If you're a young success do it right and keep it tight by staying light—that means humble not proud, meek not loud, and always stay aware from whom it came: The Lord is His name and He'll bring you acclaim. He'll cover your blame and remove your shame—let Him be your new flame.

COMPLETION OF CREATIVE ACT:

Keep getting away from it/opening up. Take the END very slowly, it's your last chance to influence pub.

BORE-DUMB

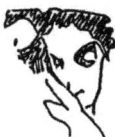

Bored-Dumb Comes From Sin. Repent:
You're No More a Has-Been as Your Life
Opens Up to Glory (Out of Trash-Bin)

When you're bored (in a world that seems so cold) all you want to do is mark time, fill time, or liven up your empty life with pleasures--but becoming a sensual devil just creates more bore-dumb. In contrast when you're excited, fascinated and enthused there's not enough minutes in the day and pleasure-seeking pales in comparison. It's important what we do when bored, lest lower lusts fill the vacuum and it's hell on earth we're going toward. The answer's always the same: dissolve obstruction, then go forward. Sometimes the only answer is to sleep and not eat—clean the cells so your senses open up and your mood becomes sweet. Now no more bored, you become hypercreative as you open to the Lord.

Bore-dumb comes from sin of act or association which blocks wide-angled perception of an abundant universe, putting one in the tunnel-vision of addiction: a gray, watered-down, fearful and bland perception of reality which makes one "dull". It's bad faith, or fullness—we can't have both, for with dulled vision we've become a bore and life becomes a chore. With flagged fascination it's third-rate having boredom as a mate.

Sin drags energy from the head to the gut or that other rut. It's like smut—it doesn't energize but just fills time as in with demons we chime. Stop, fast and pray: instantly you're ready to climb. On consciousness boredom is like a grime but repentance makes it sublime as you discover you're still in your prime! Sin puts us in the doldrums (thick slime) but by giving up the rut (not worth a dime) your new anti-crime will spice up your life (like adding thyme). Test me on this: to be happy and successful we must seek the sublime. This is maturity: making the best use of our time.

ARTS OF PALEO FASTING

BORED vs. LORD

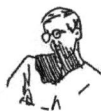

Sin steals your glory and then there's no more victory. Aren't you sick of the same old story? Be like a good child, then enter a palace all beautifully tiled. Be a little angel and don't get so riled (for anger is from sin, once beguiled). The only way to true fun and freedom from the gun is to run the good race: with acute attention to detail cover everything you do it's like your own unique creative lace. Then if you were to die today you'd leave a good trace (for sin slanders and stings like mace). Boredom occurs when the ace loses face: it closes the case, you've fallen from grace right down to the base. Then it's a case of a chase by your foes (i.e. disgrace). If you wish to keep up your pace (victory, fascination, glee) then of sin repent and Jesus says "erase"—replace the bad space for God's warm embrace. It's the aesthetic difference between filth/chaos and a beautiful vase.

WHEN YOU'RE GOOD

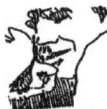

When you're good you wake-up in the arms of God and your perception takes in the whole universe: past and future unite in the pleasant moment with only fond memories of the past ("it's all been a blast"). But when bad it's a terror so vast: you've switched from constant creative revelations to the shadow figure, an outcast (you're now miscast). Do you see? Boredom won't last. It's all our past-times and associates that initiate wrong actions (when we're a donkey's ass). When you repent, bring out the brass for now you're the noble class. Remember you're living in glass (especially on the internet with gossip amassed): "what a despicable lass" they all said (the mass). But now that's all passed—"alas 'tis the empty past". What a contrast: while you were harassed (so bored) now you're unsurpassed—with your own director's board, rid of the horde, wielding a spiritual sword, with angelic accord and winning awards.

PAST AND FUTURE UNITE

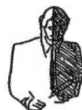

Two choices: good or bad. Being good you shoot to eternity where past and future unite. Your whole household becomes alive and you're the magic magi enlivening everyone in your charge. The pets awake (it's like a quake). Here there is no spite, you're filled with light. The mind is everywhere always—as a brilliant angel gone is the devil's bite. So end that old blight and come into the bright (it's like a flight). At this point you've ended the fight so there'll be no more fright. From lowness and boredom you've now sprung to the height, a true nobleman (a knight). Repent today and you'll have this by tonight (just do what is right). The bored are low-down and scared—"bored-white". To silence their mind they get trite (usually from getting tight). Having lost creative ideas their work is so silly and slight. That's most of Hollywood—alright? So now recite: no sin, no boredom—that's just being polite. For a moment can you be contrite? It'll be to your great delight as it will truly excite.

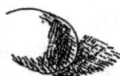

Nature just does it: the egg becomes a chicken. If you handle things right things will work out perfectly. Repent and it'll be so nice, but if in sin you'll wake-up to lice. I'll say it twice: Your life needs spice--this is true joy while sin makes ya small like mice. Why be captive to the forces of fate? For it's like rolling dice—sin freezes work like ice and that's too high of a price. So of heaven's phantasmagoria take a slice-- end that old vice. That's my good advice as I used to use the (anxiety-avoidance) device and it sure lowered my market price. I was so bored I needed sin to suffice (I had allowed it to entice). Then I was no better than beggar's lice. So I'll be concise: stop old sins and become precise.

CIRCULARITY IS CLEAR

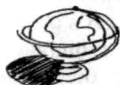

Repent, you're part of the whole universe. But the more you sin the more boring your life becomes--then you're compelled to sin more for relief from this narrow tunnel-vision. The circularity is clear and it all ends in tears. And your rep? Filled with smears. You look older (sin consumes the years), but repentance youthifies once more (to the shamed shock of your ageist-insulting peers). It was like playing musical chairs while you stayed wet behind the ears, all from having too many beers. Though encouraged by mob-cheers it strengthened your fears as that old demon interferes. Boredom blinds the mind--we seek and buy souvenirs. When bored-dumb true life disappears: Far from being pioneers we just put on airs but the bored are in arrears! Mundane and boring is how life appears if not repenting in pursuit of new frontiers. As the boredumb demon disappears some become engineers, and through repentance and prayer even great marketers.

SIN MAKES ONE BORED, UGLY AND OLD

ARTS OF PALEO FASTING

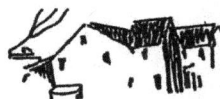

Repent and it Turns Around to Gold
Don't be like King Lear: Obsessed with getting old his life grew cold and filled with mold. I don't mean to scold but the sin life must implode if you're going for Making Gold. Just repent and let God take hold-- now you've been sold to God in the Greatest Story Ever Told. When this is over you'll say "Behold, I'm no more demon-cajoled". Through God you've been consoled so no more like the past when others controlled. Into God's arms, enfold--in the Great Mind with all the discoverers, artists and saints that ever lived you're now enrolled. That's good company with which you've been extolled, anything but this true hall of fame is fool's gold. It's a story long foretold: repent to receive a hundredfold. After being paroled are you ready to be creatively bold? This time you'll not be outsold as God takes you under His wings and begins to remold. Then your Destiny will unfold with remuneration (no more withhold).

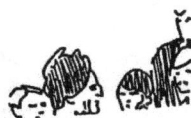

Get well, no more smell, for sin leaves a bad taste as bad memories are encased. They'll all come up as demons fill their cup. The sinner hears three successive voices: one to lasciviously swear, then one condemning him for lasciviously swearing, then the temptation to sin to deal with his guilt. These voices are wearing, while clarity is full vision under God's caring. The saints are never bored or lonely: each day, hour and minute is luxurious while the other way is spurious. It's a matter of perception—infinite immaculate conceptions of ideas, plans, goals. But with sin it's all deception: "sin is fun" is the misconception as it holds out promises, but self-deception takes no exception: our reality becomes gray and mundane as bore-dumb is sin's punishment at it's inception.

RETURN TO THE ELEMENTS AND JUST THINK

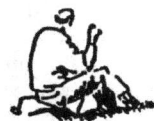

Let go of your noisy, busy senseless life and just return to the elements. This is the cure for the devil's lure. I know about all temptations (that's for sure). But when you get down, the answers lie inside if you're quiet: if you run around the brain ignores it. There is no resolution outside of you—it's all inside if you can simmer down and just enjoy the scenery all around. From such austerity comes the crown, just look at the beauty above the ground: live a charmed life as miracles abound you'll go up not down.

ANA SAGE

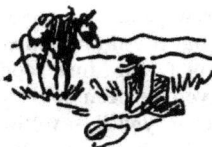

This page is for Anas and All Others Who Choose
Fasting not Swine Consciousness.

Anas are mature and recovered EDs (Eating Disorders). They possess
superior qualities characteristic of saints and genius throughout time. Ana is
a rare calling and it requires fasting to achieve it--for
only in
Fasting Consciousness
Can We See What to Do

RX: After realizing I was an obligate carnivore and told to go zero-carb I said
forget that, I'm gonna be led: In the mornings I had RAW MILK smoothies
with plain yogurt, a little coconut and nutbutter. Then I had meat then fasted
to the next day. If I ever ate in the afternoon it was just a few grapes.

PSYCHOSIS AND BULIMIA

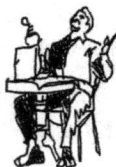

Bulimia is a secret society of not just women but men and it is
growing in leaps and bounds. This is such a massive problem and
has so many extenuating factors it becomes an obdurate and
incendiary addiction. The dialogues below are funny, tragic and
informative. In between are rational psychological explanations
from systems theory and archetypal psychiatry. The reasons for
this burgeoning pandemic are dysfunctional families and a
societal shift to wrong foods which keep the fire burning (for they create bloat
and craving). We're not eating properly anymore so the result is obesity and
feeling famished. For the vain they think the only answer is not to abstain (we
have to eat) but rather to binge and purge over and over again. It's a closet
thing and it's insane.

FASTING IS GOOD, BULIMIA IS BAD

84

ARTS OF PALEO FASTING

Question: Can you say why certain girls develop anorexia psychosa--a most serious and fatal illness?

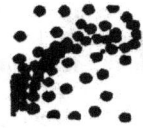

KK: Many reasons genetic, biochemical, temperamental and psycho-social (systems theory) help to set the stage. I have described the family system [Anorexic Systems] but the most powerful reason is sociobiological--survival related, to prevent death. It's genetically based they've now found: An EVENT or TRAUMA occurs then the symptoms roll out in ordered fashion. To call bulimia-psychosa hedonistic is cruelly myopic for a fatal phenomena from the early trauma creating the template: It has to do with a cerebrotonic-ectomorph (extremely sensitive) child facing unstable supplies of love, nurturance, affection or inconstant food supplies (for whatever reason) and this from the infant's perception meant certain death. Bulimia is a survival-related unconscious self-feeding device (like a ravenous beast) to "not die". This is not to blame the parents for few can understand a hypersensitive child or ectomorph (a genetic anomaly), and in this case the problem may just be an absent mother working outside the home, or in many cases the terrors of daycare or the public schools. It was for me—I was terrified from age five and feared/couldn't stand my peers, especially women who were bullies in spreading the liberal feminist narrative.

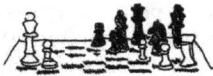

The anorexic bulimic knows she's doing it but has no idea why she *must* do it. She is eating to fill an emotional illness of EMPTINESS, but then must jettison the extra baggage in fear of losing control for she knows she's more effective "empty"—in the fasting state. Because of this fear of rejection the anorexic becomes a willing scapegoat for others' bad side--her shadow is their projection and the fear of abandonment keeps her hooked as more problems occur. She may also have had unstable supplies (nurturance) from the father either through absence, addiction or workaholism. The bulimic says "there's a hole I can't fill" and the disordered eating of gluttony (supplies for survival) and purging (separation from the suffocating system, the "vomiting up of emotions") escalates with divorce or leaving the family for college. Anorexia starts with extreme fear of abandonment coupled with a desire for independence. And yet it comes from never having totally individuated from the family system while hating it and attempting to assert independence in pathological ways. It may just be someone who is so different from the others in the system she feels terrified as the misfit from the pack. If she be a hypersensitive (to their chemicals, smoking etc) she is further singled out.

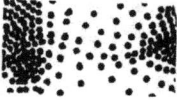

She wants to individuate but that takes having been nurtured consistently in the first place so instead she feels suffocated and starts to separate, but then the fears of emotional immaturity relapses back into pathology. Due to the absent or indifferent father template she may become promiscuous or even morally insane which is now called "borderline" (using sex to prevent rejection, which happens anyway) though her true nature is the opposite--that of marriage to God, purity, celibacy and a monastic life in total faith in her divine (father) provider. She is searching for her divine Protector but in humans meets disastrous disappointment. The original peace was invaded by hostile elements (to the soul or the temperament) to whose control she reacts by "sex for approval". A bulimic slut is a mutt but it's all over the minute she seals the gut, makes gold and refuses their mean projections (becomes Queen Tutt). The anorexic is a driven perfectionist so if she can just survive the system and habit she can shoot to the top (a divine strut).

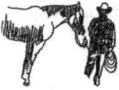

A woman or girl caught in this early template will often have extreme affections for animals while avoiding people for whom she has strange unexplained antipathies. She'll have uncontrolled rages and depressions, inner voices (from past introjects) bringing guilt and shame, detailed memories of sibling put-downs (though occurring decades back by siblings who have no memory of them), obsessions with people and an ongoing feeling of rejection. The answer for this unfortunate victim of herself, society and circumstances is to fast and revel in solitude (come to herself, dissolve distorted implants).

Question: My gosh, that's heavy! Did this happen to you?

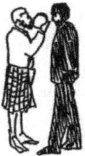

KK: Yes—I was raised by a wonderful Scotchman but then alcoholism infected the home and it became a conspiratorial climate—a hostile environment with harassing Hitlerian harridans in control. As the father receded I lost emotional support and became a mindless robot caught up in a sociobiological template enslaved to a habit just to survive. Only fasting and solitude set me free to find and be me, and now it's not food I need for survival but fasting and selfhood free of obstruction and continuous closeness to my true Father God upon whom I rely for everything. The Ana Angel with a Black Eye must deal with her hypersensitivity in a cruel cold world: "to be a world rage, escape this cage". To me that means land, a fence and a locked gate.

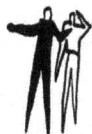

"Karen, thanks so much for "Anorexic Systems" [Champion Guides]. It feels so good when there's someone who understands. I'm a Brazilian bulimic and now I feel liberated from this destructive cycle which I don't want anymore--but it's so hard to overcome the feelings of rejection. Every time there's a hint of it in the air I feel like binging. But now I'm aware and hope to begin a new phase..."

To all victims of a terrible illness, but not if managed correctly:

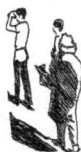

When we stop in-filling the big hole inside, and make gold, we open up in full fidelity to what is now perceived as an abundant environment and every moment becomes rich and fascinating. I'd do anything to keep this going because I know that if in sin one loses all interest like this, the magic cornucopia of everyday life. The recovered ED fills his life with more life, not feed an empty hole.

REJECTION

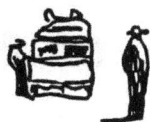

Most anas felt rejected by family, love or conformist society. Rejection anxiety triggers binging to relieve anxiety which brings on more rejection--and therein is the self-destructive cycle of the negative ana life-phase. Fasting not binging is the way to break the cycle raising self-esteem, regaining confidence and beauty and forgiving the rejecters. Those rejecters have always loomed large but now their huge significance dissolves (the fast broke through this obstructive barge if living with a sarge).

DISCUSSION

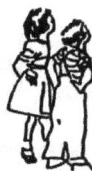

Ana 1: Karen I so agree with your analysis above. If I may recap all you've said: Due to our rare hypersensitivity we never felt nurtured so we couldn't properly individuate, yet feel suffocated and imposed upon from the outside. Bulimia gives us that (seeming) nurturance, but then it ruins us so we become ashamed (dependent) again (shame allows others to take control). We have so many conflicts: eating to nurture ourselves but not eating not to

depend, hating what we see projected onto us but accepting these horrible intrusions to be loved. It's a conflict between needing love but hating the kind of love we're getting. In the past I remember trying to be accepted in groups I hated. And until I read you I was tied to my rejecters! We can't stand rejection but we can't stand intrusion. It's so painful as these conflicts constantly throw us back to that uncomfortable place in our infancy. And in order to be an individual rejection fears must be released and since this is impossible we end up alone--and this is heaven as all conflicts solved. What a life--but as you say if we thank God for this life we see all the bounty coming from it! Thank you for saving my life from all this strife. I'm happily a daily faster now eating fat like a cat--and all this crap is over just like that!

KK: That is a perfect restatement.

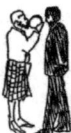

Ana 2: I never heard of an anorexic who was not bulimic. I guess it all comes from not feeling safe as a child so we learned to nurture ourselves—with insults food fullness makes us feel a loss of control (vulnerable) so we have to jettison the obstruction. KK: Our people problems (the cerebrotonic usually ending the system-scapegoat) isolate us completely and though we know what is happening we feel powerless—unless fasting. And since we want love (and status in hostile systems) we become thin-perfectionists (since the world sees that as superior and we feel so strong when thin) which nevertheless becomes a pathological cycle--though it never works we keep trying. By the world this is viewed as vanity by (usually fat) women who become very abusive to the thin female, which just magnifies the rejection problem. So there's a conflict: they need to eat, they need to binge--but they also need a perfect body and image and to regain control so they purge. The anorexic-bulimic life is a constant fight between these two needs. We must see we can never get unconditional love from humans but desire thinness (in purity) just because it's fun. The fast (after fueling with fat or fruit) is the only way to break the chains. And the bulimic never gains, it just leaves stains. P.S. If she eats veggies she hates the "truck in her gut".

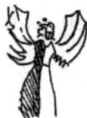

Karen: All I think about is food and cravings. But I want to be a daily fastarian, having it be my whole life. How do I get over the hump? KK: I know all about cravings and food obsession, the desire to eat everything in the universe. Only by eating fat can you overcome this—daily fat-fasting is your answer. Have raisins when first hungry--that is the Grapecure. Then, have a fatty meal like doughless pizza or cheese omelet. Better yet--for awhile, just eat the omelet and delete all sugar to attain complete stability, calmness and moist skin. Now you can easily fast without ever thinking about food until the next morning or longer. Each day you are cleaner (as the eliminative system takes over) and have greater self-restraint. Giving into desire was on your personality a severe taint. This will dissolve your cravings for there is nothing more delicious and with fat needs met, the craving is gone. Now that you have your obsession under control read the ten books during your fasting afternoons to make you more receptive.

Karen: It feels so good to write out the system and my extreme emotions on it. I started to fast then suddenly after a lifetime of sister-abuse I saw the system and rejected it for good. I saw her subtle cruel sarcasm--and realized I had been back-stabbed for 30 years! I feel so good--so incredibly good to have finally transcended the system that held me down--is this not my "Separation-Unto-the-Highest-Calling Event"?

KK: Yes, that's always the way--the victim is blamed for the very thing the other has always done then the anorexic keeps purging up the system. It's a mindless trap but when suddenly this scene is seen you're free--you've won. Enantiodromia has occurred—now who's preferred? When you're rich you have relatives coming out of the floor. When you're poor they'll show you the door.

Karen: I ate an apple yesterday and woke up complete groggy and unable to think. What happened?

KK: Insulin spike. We so ravaged our metabolisms from years of promiscuous eating and purging from multi-combinations of foods that our immunity was suppressed so now all fruit causes an insulin spike--low blood sugar, fatigue, brain fog, next day craving. I have found the dried black fruit is a slow spike--it just cleans and nourishes--but juicy fruit gets in the blood fast--we crash. Most bulimic anorexics end up on purely lowcarb high fat dieting, and they become slim, trim, fit, peppy and filled with wit.

Karen: Can you please elaborate on sister struggles?

ARTS OF PALEO FASTING

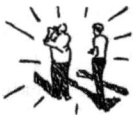

KK: Such identity struggles are basic to systems theory. We get our identity *in relation to others* in the family system. One can only be seen as "superior" if the "inferior" stays that way and thus these identity struggles get very cruel since maintaining identity is *basic*. Oh, the joys of going beyond this problem—to cosmic perception! But with low self-esteem (from addiction) they become survival struggles to the death, accounting for the horrors of homelife in the lives of the ungodly. The Godly in contrast get their identity from God--they know He has a destiny and purpose for them alone and thus they lose the competitive struggle since they are defined by God, not vis-à-vis other members of the family. Sick systems seek only to maintain themselves while healthy systems evolve or dissolve.

Ana: Beyond the systems dynamic of anorexia which you describe so shockingly well, what about the binging (swine) consciousness? I feel I will never go beyond it. I keep eating all day, sinking into despair.

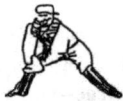

KK: I understand—you get well you must be a catcher of all evil thoughts and associations. Become alert to cruel sting-shots and flip-flops—for though you may be blind they still register subconsciously and drill holes in your gut (the basis of your rut). You must become an "anger-detective". See the signs: subtle sarcasm, sullen sudden silence, not responding, and dyads and triads rising up against you (triangulation-strangulation). I have to constrain to one fatty meal, then fly off to a high-bliss fast to be ready for the crass (who want to miscast me) and nevertheless have a blast. It is good for you to realize how different anas are: birdlike engines who just can't take more than one meal (other than a mouse-meal of fruit later to cleanse out all residue). We gotta stay high or die. Being ana we can't try certain things anymore. We must realize who we are and act accordingly. It's not easy to not-eat--to not be oral--but the refusal to give in blasts out all previous neurotic circuitry, and now we are free. At first it seems like nothingness, a vast terrifying void but soon God fills it with bliss-- the new life's in view, we're coming to the crest. For anas it's a rare responsibility: transcend the body or succumb to the horrors of normal living. We must relish our own separate ana reality. It's a matter of what happens when we eat: confusion, critical mass. The day becomes "empty"-- we lack *fullness of experience* and become a blank field feeling senseless and bored (being floored by the barbarian horde). The energy has leaked from the brain to the gut from being in the same old rut. With more maturity these episodes become intolerable for we see the destruction they create—more with time and age.

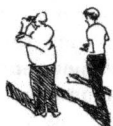

The other sin we commit is self-disgust because the world is disgusted. We can't live in cosmic perception due to continuous guilt and shame--most of us are system-lame. We may have lost our families and friends (and we know why) but forget it—for now we're high as the sky. The Bible says all men are sinners--there are no winners. Who points a finger at the lone anorexic? The fornicator, the adulterer, the whoremonger, the drunk, the gambler, the liar or the gossiper. All through history the fornicating male community disdained the sins of the females--usually food problems. Everyone's a sinner but their sins are socially-condoned while those of the lonely ana are not. So we took on the shame, the image-rot. It was a terrible burden: the results of our rare make-up spoiled the entire lot. But if we overcame it and recover we became the best and win the whole pot.

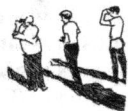

Avoid self-disgust or you'll rust. It's time to do your work or bust—attract others to your new cornucopic perception! Thank God each morning you are given another chance: new life. Each dawn is a new beginning so forget the past (even if you slipped last night) and try again, soon you'll get it right. You want a slim and strong body, vivid lucid perception, keen discernment, energy to work all day (starting before dawn) and total success in this era—all on one meal a day (OMAD) and I recommend FAT, animal that is, blood gold.

Karen: I feel so out of place like I'm from another planet. It makes me want to eat everything in sight. Please help me .

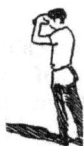

KK: I understand! All through youth I felt out of place--it was a pain in the solar plexus (stomach), a cry stuck in my throat, a terror and "school phobia" or "sunday school phobia" or "church retreat phobia" and later "sorority phobia"--it was all what I call "peer-phobia". Later it was fear of my sisters, they had changed so much in college (and I had gone in reverse) it produced an ontologically fatal insight that became terror, pain, dread, fright. This unexplainable terror became alcoholism and anorexia--anything to "shut up" the feelings. I would seek older people but these systems would degenerate too, for the real problem was separation from the True Self and God. It led me to write for as I matured I saw many misfits--and especially genius--die of addictions used to quiet these out of sync feelings. If you can find a way to revel in your solitude--to love and adore your own home life and develop your talents you will be fine and skip the dark decades I dragged through, not knowing. You'll transcend people with this diet plan since you'll forget all about food (your past mal-adaptation to intruders) and the struggle will be gone. When first hungry I fix my raw milkshake with plain yogurt, nut butters and coconut. It's delicious and satiating and then I have my meal. I'm done with eating by 9 am and now revel in the exciting no-food day that lies before me. You'd be surprised to know how lucid it all is once food is removed.

Ana: Karen, I sometimes drink a lot for days. I lose all control and start calling for confirmation.

KK: I did it for years thinking drinking was revving up the day then telephonitis would set in. The next morning I'd wake up so ashamed I'd start drinking again. I finally realized that it was turning the light OFF, not ON. Instead of wide-angled perception I just became a shadow misconception standing in my own light. Demons were waiting for (luring) me to drink so they could work through me—I see this now in retrospect, the drinking years were in the pit of hell. The antithesis was sober ana consciousness, sweet and enduring as we enjoy each pithy moment. To have that wonderful state we must see worldly things like alcohol for what they are—devil entrapment, turning your life off. Forget all the pro-wine sites—just enjoy grape juice. Anas may relapse into this dark dungeon and telephonitus sets in because they're isolated and feel rejected anyway. Revel in your solitude--that's the way to transcend the world who eats food and avoid drinking (and other crude things).

TRUE DIVERSITY

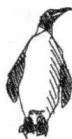

When first opening up I became multi-cultural: black and white and everything in between. Having separated from the limitations of my origins I was exhilarated with newfound energy as I explored all cultures. In horror of the strange brutalities and coarseness of other peoples I escaped back into good ol' Americana and human rights like saying what I want with the right to defend myself. The New Tolerance is an evil thing. However as boundaries break down between you and the entire *animal* kingdom it's different--you begin a charmed life of continuous miracles.

ARTS OF PALEO FASTING

Ana: What do you think of television?

KK: It's strange because I pay for TV but never turn it on. I don't want to take what I'm served but decide where I go every minute. I don't want my mind to be tracked, I am constantly turning everything off to return to center.

Ana: I feel sequestered by my two sisters--they go off without me and I'm always the odd man-out.

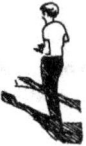

KK: Another template obstructing your cosmic view, this happened to me too. Most cruelty comes from identity-management: The opinion-leaders of the clan (two older sisters) dissuade their progeny against the dissident who is isolated against the pronounced sense of extended family with her excluded, and primitive anas feel this incredibly deeply. Evolved anas however will be unaffected, even relieved. All the nieces and nephews have been educated to exclude/hate/ridicule. It's like being a Jew in Nazi Germany: the daily acts of exclusion become a habit--and children can be cruel! To avoid her is the family rule. It hurts--it's just not cool. But if it doesn't kill her it perfects her when out of the family zoo (for only this is true). Is she ready to transcend the system so her emotions won't be their tool? I've written of the Ana Sister System or Cinderella Syndrome, let this be your school.

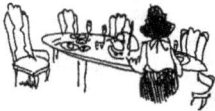

We live in a culture of extreme female competition and Cinderella is ageism in reverse—the older may hate the younger. The older siblings can't admit the superiority of the younger so their cruel exclusions are used for identity maintenance. Female bullies fight through *exclusion*, not fists. To stabilize their fragile identity they must collude together to find her flaws and no matter how trivial they blow it up (they show their claws). This becomes a vicious system as the younger in trying to prove herself triggers even more rejection, then more need for proof (they call her a spoof, she hits the roof). This drives her into more striving for perfection until they reject her altogether. When we change, old systems lose their comfort zone and it's a really bad tone. But it's ok since at this point she now has world success instead (if she passes the test of letting them go--dropping the lead: the walking dead). Many solitary anas end up alone but look up for this frees them to the highest calling--the eagle has finally left the chicken coop and the second

ARTS OF PALEO FASTING

half of life is wonderful compared to the first half which was miserable (being marginal to the troop). Now that she's transcended the system she feels cool.

Ana: That is so fascinating--the lasting though delusional effects of sick systems! What makes you so poetic? And what is the biggest myth of the medical profession?

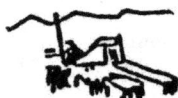

KK: Let the old system become a silly ghost town in mind. Poetry is not a statement of emotion so much as a way of dealing with emotions. I learned it was better to elicit reactions through the subtle rather than describe the war— that only made readers sore. Poetry or picture-strips, we all have different bents. It comes naturally so I think God wants me to intersperse text with verse and imagery. People don't learn from long treatises and science journals but from hidden analogies in short quips. Suddenly they reverse matrices and see the whole, that's my role.

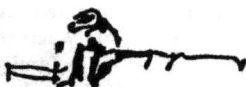

The biggest myth of the medical profession is that anas can ever eat "normally". No way we can be happy with a truck in the gut—all those fermenting fibrous vegetables and grains. The meat melts right in, our deficiencies relieved, power and nutrients flood our being. Dry skin gone, complexion smooth as porcelain. No defiencies, no family complain. The ana living my way will look a child at ninety (much like Ghandi).

Ana: Karen your advice is perfect. The fact is we anas cannot eat in the traditional sense. For me, a regular meal is pure hell. It's a bite here, one there and that's IT. Our only goal is to kill the hunger. Ana is not something you choose--it is something you are--in my opinion, a blessing from God. He has put this "thing" in us--the Ana calling--and with that has made us allergic to food. Before we realize this, however, we may fall into bulimia and this becomes the obstacle we must overcome. To anas I would say "reject bulimia for good, but don't fight your good ana tendencies--embrace it and rejoice. You are special."

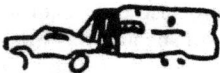

KK: Right! Just like celibacy is a personal calling also fasting, or daily fastarianism, is. The fact that promiscuous disordered eating has never worked must tell us something—it can start us on our lifelong vacation if we watch that ration. Let me try to rhyme: I don't dare eat more than my one fatty meal, or it starts the bad ana process (I reel). Shrink the gut to a walnut--that's my even keel. I won't even try to eat "normally" again--that's my spiel. To bulimic anas longing for new life: be a mature recovered anorexic. Eating is just our fuel for the whole day so that we may re-enter the fast which is our blast. We eat fat to make it last.

Ana: Aren't we supposed to have a little more variety, like everyone says?

KK: Not necessarily, I don't mind monotony for simplicity marks all traditional living. In the old frontier they went to town for bacon (etc.) and coffee once a month. My present routine is morning raw milkhake then chicken or fish then fast. Simple, kitchen stays clean and sparse. Not a bunch of things around cuz we're confused and always on the search. We've found what prevents the hearse. But you must pre-decide exactly what works for you. Suggestions: Nut-butters, grapes/raisins, lemons, lettuce, nuts, cheese and eggs, canned fish, pineapple and olives, clean top fish or chicken breasts for the freezer. Now just relax and enjoy your life of prolific work output and much time-saving from the superfluity of most kitchens and food life.

Ana: I agree about mono-diet. One time I ate navel oranges for 30 days and was so high! I could never understand why everyone else bought so much variety in foods. At least we should just eat one thing at a time, then fast for as long as possible and then eat one thing again. Eating should always be just "breaking the fast" and if we restrict to just one thing we automatically cut down. Variety makes us hungry for different flavors....

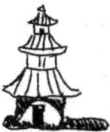

KK: Even that is too rulish for me. Just follow the break-fast program and all will fall into perfect place. Many of these rules will fall by the wayside. Variety leads to food-obsession, simplicity leads to fasting consciousness and bliss—viva la France, we start to prance! The more mono your foods the more macro your experience. The more mono ("boring") your food life the most fascinating your perceptual life and soon food falls out of thought altogether since the bodymind knows it's gonna be fed once a day. The truth is life is infinitely more fascinating and satisfying--lushly varied--without food and all other lower lusts. Nothing ages you faster--it means rust. You must now think "youthification or bust."

Ana: You're right Karen. Variety leads to food obsession for us hypersensitive anas and that is not what we are about. Keep it simple and it'll keep you light.

ARTS OF PALEO FASTING

SUPERIOR PALEO-FASTERS NOT ANAS

Question: Can you distinguish between good and bad anorexia, and do you feel anorexics are superior? KK: Anas are a separate class with a special calling based on finding God and the True Self. They need privacy to do this, by being set apart and fasting. Since women base their identity by how well they do socially vis-à-vis female culture, this can be a very rocky trip. Many die from suicide or drugs, feeling inferior because they don't "fit". But God has set us apart—separation means "holy" so just persevere, enjoy it and succeed (stay lit).

Ana: Ok so Ana's are elite yet envied and misunderstood? KK: Ana is not Karen Carpenter but rather Arnold Ehret. In fact Ana's as a group are much healthier than the population at large and will outlive them as well. Anorexia is not a "diet" or a disease. It is a way of life: restricted and disciplined for a greater calling. Unfortunately today there are many "pro-ana" websites which distort the true meaning: short on maturity and knowledge they steal from others what might have been an anointed life through the miracle of solitude. But faint not--for you are not out to change the world--only yourself.

ANA DISCUSSION
with a Binge-Recoveree

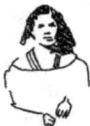

Ana: I'm only happy fasting. Eating disgusts me. I want my life to mean something. I don't see how I can possibly do that and live a life of eating. Meals? I cringe at the thought. Sure I may graze, but never do I sit down to a meal. And the family system? It is competitive. I feel diminished as my parents favor my sisters. But I am learning from you to purposely be "small", like a Saint. Ana is more than just food, though eating makes one mean, ugly, bitter and fasting makes us a calm, restful sea. It's about just being quiet--the kind, selfless little anorexic. Don't talk about yourself--just watch from the sidelines and remain invisible as you do your work and find your gifts.

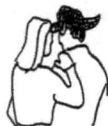

KK: Ana goes way beyond eating, doesn't it? It hits the painful cobwebs of human systems imposing on us. So the saints acted little"--inconsequential, expecting nothing. Get into expecting nothing from people but the sky's the limit from God! Yes being a Saint is the only way to survive the sick system in which you are devaluated--often just because you're a girl. Take heart--your family problems only indicate your ana status. Revel in it. Be proud of it. It's all in the way you look at it which determines the outcome. Just don't ever slip into the bad characteristics like purging—if you do that your family has every right to drop the bad apple out of the cart.

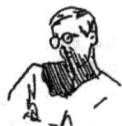

Had you fasted rather than binged at the situation yesterday you'd have felt totally different. Fasting attracts everything to you, and "acting small" triggers adoration. Humility works but ego shows your quirks. Whenever in an odd-man-out situation, fast--and you'll see positive results; vs. utter devastation resulting from eating or drinking *at* it. Yes, by being little we're bigger than life. Everyone else is talking, gossiping, self-revealing so by us being little and silent we stand out like a thumb while they look dumb. Ego is unattractive and it makes others reactive. Obviously we cannot compete in the world of big men and manly women. This is the only way to compete--and only the saints (knowing they are backed by God--the Biggest) know the secret info that *less is more.* Dying to self is the beginning of new life for being little or nothing makes us everything--to them and to God who rewards us with power and glory. Just wait and see! And incidentally, don't ever expect them to agree with you that your disease is an adaptation to them (or the warped liberal narratives coming *through* them).

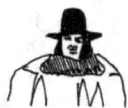

Ana: These writings are my guide, my sanity in this ana world and terrible eating ordinary society. No one else talks about these things! When nothing makes sense, I read your words and suddenly everything makes sense. Nothing matters yet you make everything matter. I have learned to stop fighting the system and just be the little sweet anorexic who cares about others and doesn't talk about herself to them. To rise above and just "love the little evil children"--the immature adults around me, "steeped in silly stereotypes" as you say. I love it when you say "had you fit your family (been accepted), you'd be ordinary--fat, ugly, bitter, mean, materialistic, hungry, stupid and petty." ha ha ha ha--I love your wit, thank God for your wit--so many times you took me out of the depths of suicidal depression.."

ARTS OF PALEO FASTING

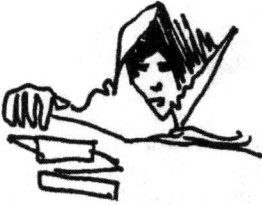

KK: If one does not know God, being demeaned triggers demonic fixes and yes, your binges are triggered by family visits. Pin-point the specific triggers for you, for whatever reason: good, bad, right or wrong. It's your template: *reactive food devices*. If you feel your sister is their favorite it makes you heart-sick and the automatic response is to eat (cheat, peep, tweak) to self-medicate, to self-nurture since no one else will. You can't help yourself blindly caught in the template but now you're no longer blind—so I hope I'm not unkind when I say we must repent, and not just for lent. The power of the template can be broken by *just one time* fasting at the system rather than *eating* at it. As you learn how fasting at this trigger works better you'll break the automatic response (brain grooves) while also forgiving and loving your family. But most books on anorexia are about food as no one can imagine the cure is to fast--that is inconceivable. All therapy is about the anorexics "eating normally" and what a cold nightmare to be part of it.

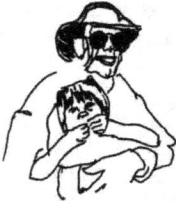

Ana: I just want the happiness of childhood—guess that's why I love children but in this era we can't get too close lest we be accused. KK: We all want childhood vitality but it's like cocaine: the first hit is great but increasingly you're third rate. It's now all about food and the "raw food crowd"—a social party where we feel crappy so buy their superfoods to be healthy. If you ask me they aren't childlike but rather neurotic adults. I feel most cornucopic (childlike) when I eat fauna and then fast. As long as we think it's all about food--this food, or that--we are forever eating and wasting time with recipes and "uncooking" shows. It's so simple and this is needlessly complex! Just do your work and forget all this. Thaw you a steak, eat it, and forget it. NOW you have "found time" to work. I arise at 2 am and work until 5 pm—that's a 15 hour day even on Sundays. Women have to work ten times harder than men so with perseverence they end with a masterpiece bassed on acute attention to detail, everything perfect—so isn't it all worth it?

Ana: I keep re-reading your "Fast Miracles"--a fine piece of work! I have to start my fasting miracles diary, and realize that fasting at the trigger *always* works, and eating at it *never* works. I will keep reminding myself every day, so I'll be ready when the system switches into negative gear (again). I can't believe how eating at this is such an automatic response. Now that I know better I can work extra hard at it. Nobody said ana was easy. I have to start fasting at my family instead of hating them. They'll never change who they like best--but that doesn't mean I have to sit and feel horrible for it when I could feel good for fasting, right? KK: Yes in order to live comfortably in the disconfirming system you must transcend it, looking down on the poor dumb enviers of your soul. This may help during the inevitable *pre-success crisis*:

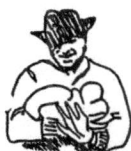

SLOGANS FOR ANAS TO HANG ONTO WHEN PRE-SUCCESS CRISES ABOUND:

Before triumph comes tribulation.

Endure, avoid lure, take cure.

I will bless those who bless you and curse those who curse you

Promotion is not from the east or the west. God is the judge--He puts one up just as He puts the other down [it's a moral test]

Those who forsake the law praise the wicked. Those who keep the law forsake them. Both he who condemns the just and he who loves the wicked are an abomination to the Lord.

Man wants the approval of man, but beware if everyone speaks well of you. For the world hated Me before they hated you.

Intolerance of your present condition creates your future. What you are willing to walk away from determines what God will take you to.

They shall gather together--but not by Me. I shall condemn every voice that rises against you.

☐

ARTS OF PALEO FASTING

LIFE:
my only responsibilities

1. Love God and be open to His inspirations

2. Take good care of pets and any one under my charge

3. Keep perfect house (create a spiritual/fascinating environment)

4. Sequence the music correctly, grouping for moods

5. Stay neat and attractive

6. Keep household well-supplied with good (not bad) things

buying bulk of a simple list.

7. Be a good hostess but vet all visitors.

Hi Karen,

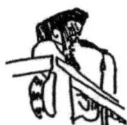

Dear Karen I feel wonderful living this way. I have my main meat meal in the morning then a couple grapes if anything before bed. The food thoughts and cravings are gone and now all dry skin has vanished. I am so surprised but what surprises me more than anything is how my friends have 86ed me for being "cruel".

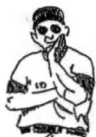

KK: This is a time to reflect on all we've learned so far: What we should want is youthification for that opens all doors. At any age that's the goal and that's what daily fasting does--for youthification is simply mysticism, and that comes from being mature, showing them the door! I see "youth" as well as elderhood as a combo of mysticism, infantilization and what looks like to them as psychosis but is in fact our own (cornucopia of the right-brain). I'm happy to lose my reality every day since that opens new doors as creative insight outpours.

This is the
CHILD POWER-STATE

comes from daily fasting after eating right:
fruit or fauna fat.

ARTS OF PALEO FASTING

NEVER SITTING DOWN,
THE CLOWN
Non-Egotism

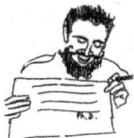

Now you'll be the opposite to the egotistic crowd who's always boasting and bragging. To be sweetly (non-ego) never be seen eating, or taking a chance that an unexpected visitor may find you eating. How disgusting--we must remain above all this as fastarians. Why not just equip the house with things that require no preparation or refrigeration--that is trail mix (make it yourself, choosing exactly the dry fruit and nuts you want)). Other than that have your fauna meal in the morning before business hours so you can transcend the herd all day long in the fasting state. Simple. He whose energy is above the gut during business hours wins hands down.

FAST-REPENT FOR DIVINE VINDICATION
Relieving Thoughts

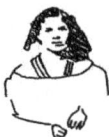

Do you have backstabbing, belittling relatives? Well get ready for the Big Payback! Soon you'll see it as fact for God's revenge is necessary for the relief of the Saints, as proof that God is just. To think otherwise brings aging cynicism—you rust. Those sting-shots and flip-flops brought constant stress (as recurrently, your joys combust). Abuse gave you thorns as it formed an ugly crust. But fast-repentance dissolves this induced-schizophrenia from others (distorted implants and templates) which blocked success through self-disgust. Recall always our slogan: All men are sinners, your accusers are filled with lusts. See much of your exhaustion as the result of oppression—letting inferiors in to rain on your parade (you got jade), and take the wind out of your sails (God heard your wails). Now recovered, you can forgive them all so your resentments are smothered. Through forgiveness your mind and thoughts are mothered.

EVIL HELPERS
Words of Caution to the Cute

Trust God not the clod. God give em the rod-- I can
forgive but sure wanna forget 'em-- the mob

ARTS OF PALEO FASTING

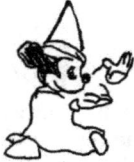

The Devil's trying to hold the cute down and he's doing it through people so you must stay high like a steeple. If not they'll make you feeble, isn't that incredible? It's as sure as dogs eating kibble--the herd seeks to slay and win the metal. Unholy ties abound so they begin to meddle. Watch out for evil helpers who betray like Judas. Inside you hate the treachery but denial puts you in mush-mode mentally. You cannot create amidst constant betrayal: I don't mean to be rude but it was with your life they screwed. Reptiles are weak and will rip your life like a knife. Don't forget Selena killed by a jealous helper in strife. I invite you to look back to those times where fear and supposed need for protection attracted an evil helper into your life. Relying on people is a sign of lost faith in God, the only Giver of success and wealth. If you can give up these heavy useless burdens (who come late, miss your date and keep you confused--third rate) you'll be flying high like the stealth.

RECLUSE PRAYER

Lord, give me Your best. Since it's better than I   could ever conceive, give me rest. No guilt--to You I confessed.   No worry--that's my test. No competition for I'm at my crest.

For success you must have: solitude, sobriety
and no silly friends (silence)

Tell your casual drop-ins to
"Stop Talking and Just Listen to the Music".

Shine while you can
LET GOD LIFT YOU UP
to prosper and succeed

"You did not choose me--I chose you out of the
world to bear much fruit, for you are

Destined for Greatness

marked before the Foundations of the Earth..."

GLAMOROUS AGING
The True Lady is Gentle Worldliness, not Worldly Grossness

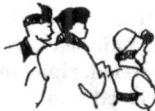

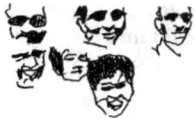

Glamorous aging is growing into your own skin— becoming more yourself as the years pass. This is magnetic, charismatic and perfect. It's like finding a brand new life as a five year old—totally spontaneous and creative. As you clear up from false roles each moment will be blissful, flamboyant and lucid with new sights and sounds. The glamorous elder's days are packed-in with ecstatic enjoyment—intense happiness after so much pain and distress. To partake of this bliss *remove the obstructions* and get ready for transformation--a striking alteration in appearance and character. Though so many years have passed you're younger than you were before the fast.

RESURRECTING UNLIVED LIFE

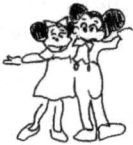

To adapt and become an "adult" we sacrificed parts of self, but now in midlife these longings scream for attention--giving into them is the joy of midlife transformation. It is a wonderful paradox that it is facing death (*thanatos*) that brings completion (success) or midlife career change. But only by first releasing the phony social image can we become the explorer, the creative child, the student or public voice that speaks out—and finally have clout. When ignored these betrayed voices go underground, hushed by constant TV, loud sounds or seeking the town. But when we *fall out of time structure* it all comes to the surface, starving for attention. Having refused the call of destiny (choosing the outer over the inner) now's the time to complete its call. If we can't do this we should shift awareness to the hidden blessings in the path we took—seeing there could not have been any other way. Seeing things this way

103

will relieve you more than you'll ever know—from cowering small you'll now walk tall.

LIFE REVIEW

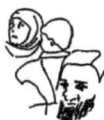

Eldering is re-assembling life in these three parts: recontextualizing, forgiving and reclaiming unlived life. In so doing we can see the unique character, charm and meaning of our own life despite the weird, ridiculous and "unforgivable" things we did. Most of us received "hot potatoes" from the people shaping our original templates—in judgments, fears and restraints—which in turn shaped our (often absurd) behavior. In eldering we forgive it all while going deeper to examine the template, change its form and then release the grudges. It is amazing how everything is seen in reverse, how the sordid and horrifying becomes pleasant and wholesome through new eyes. Older, I'm higher than the skies--even seeing the good in family spies.

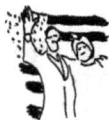

This wonderful view-reversal re-connects us to nature and God, bringing great joy and relief. Through this elder expansion (EE) we see our own unique life as created by God to enhance our Seed Symbol (of the true self) and make us strong. It's a wonderful global awareness which instantly releases cynical depression, and what a joyous experience--accepting the inevitable *rightness* of how events unfolded, marveling at the living work of art we've become as the spirit completes us. *No matter what, it was right.* Even that night we got tight? Yes, for it brought out the spite, so as we woke-up in fright we called on God's might then became a sprite. Wasted decades? No way, for these circuitous paths taught us the most. No matter how bleak and painful they created the perfect stew—who we are today, the highest display.

FROM CULTURAL STEREOTYPES TO UNIVERSAL ARCHETYPES

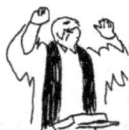

When we were young we let false churchists and phony groups create reality, telling us what is "real", our joy to steal, blocking what we could feel. Losing our own reality made us reel for these distorted implants bashed the joy of the inner life. So now we're better off solo with just a few people with whom we interact. Taking on the reality of other people (without knowing it, for we were young) was hell—we no longer rang a bell. On our personality it left a smell. We can't be someone else for they have their history and we have ours. So was life a waste of hours? No way—it took what it took to get to today. Now is the time for the True Self to really alight, as we substitute silly, sullen negative cultural stereotypes of aging for positive universal archetypes of great dignity, bearing and deep understanding.

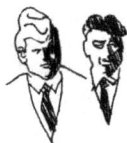

To get to the joyous universal, give up on the cultural. In universal fairytales, age brings the richness of True Maturity, in which our inner amplitude—receptivity to the moment—gets deeper. Wow—to just stare off into space and have so much happening in the mind, what a find. I can hardly believe the utter depth and richness of each moment and day. In this state, the painful past collapses and the moment—containing both past and future— becomes "pithy" with rich meaning. Now compare this with the cultural view of aging: narrowed vision, uselessness, disease and lost meaning. Never identify with cultural stereotypes, only universal archetypes for all cultures are sick to a degree, and only the transcendent is richly relevant human experience.

BELLE AGING: TRUE SEXINESS

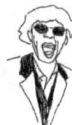

Universal aging ("oriental aging") is a positive increase into more meaningful wholes. I call this *belle aging*, meaning increased beauty and "rings a bell" wisdom: We ring-a-bell in the collective unconscious through universal archetypes recognizable to all. This is true dignity: having cut away all superfluous elements (culture-race-gender) from the core the True Self becomes *not less but more.*   We are belle-gorgeous, belle-recognized though never seen before. We become the   "well-known unknown"--a unique one-time-in-life event. It's no loud-mouth uncouth—it's the "I" as a symbol of eternity, an image encrypted on the moon. Belle aging is a sage getting better every day with no envy of youth but instead reveling in true life's mystery as a sleuth.   Facing death frees us of the major blocks-- guilts and shames—and so the elder is "grand": a joy to be around as he helps others through the shame and guilt from being youthfully outer-directed (being bound).

PERSONAL FIREPOWER: "AGELESS ALLURE"
Pure Not the Lure

ARTS OF PALEO FASTING

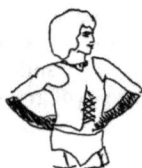

The pure hate the sex lure. Gorgeous belle aging comes from personal firepower: the explosive vibes out-dazzling mere anatomy making age irrelevant. Belle aging is pure personality built through years and character--rarified charm, a special presence growing with the years. True "sexiness" has nothing to do with age unless one defines "sexy" in the most stereotyped and boring way--superficially or culturally. Sexiness is personality and character not prowess like lower animals ("studs"). Sex has little to do with this aura of sexuality but rather a rare charm written on the face through the years, a hard-won aura which took time like fine wine.

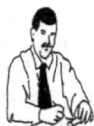

Take the ageless allure of older movie idols seducing the world through the camera. With age their special presence grows, not dims for as masters of their crafts they're at the top of their game—and masterful men are very sexy. The paradox of their charisma is the lack of super-sexuality: Cary Grant's muscles never gleamed but his wit did as subtlety was his style. He gave "fun" a high status and in it's proper form fun is rare. Innocent subtlety is an achievement of time. Having witnessed evil and vulgarity the elder increasingly chooses the purely refined—dry wit not the gross pits--George Burns, not Howard Sterns. Is there anything more disgusting, a man pushing sixty mimicking that lewd dude? Wake-up boomers—with the crude have your feud.

MATURITY IS BEST, FOR IT HAS ZEST

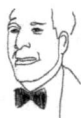

When our perceptions change in elderhood we become filled with energy. And this limitless zest doesn't wane for who else but the elder makes well-being so attractive, rarely succumbing to self-pity? These aged humans are never boring but have an infinite capacity for surprise. More growth, more zest—until just before death they're on the crest. We must grow as ageless children or pay more for remaining the neurotic phony "adult." The mature man learns to ceaselessly dare, setting out on new adventures with the manic energy of youth but with consistent excellence, fascination, experimentation. Though not eternally young he's eternally ageless triumphantly growing into his own skin. No one's ever bored in his presence. When aged, nothing dulls his appeal for he has a right to it as one who relates to spirit—his own and God's.

SUPREME SELF-CONFIDENCE

ARTS OF PALEO FASTING

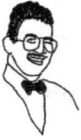

The older human knows when to talk, when not to and when not to argue with a lush or a louse. As ego recedes he has learned not to fight but to rise *above*. He tries not to provoke and has learned the fine art of walking away gently. Having transcended cultural stereotypes he sees *across* race/gender lines. He's of the world—he can truly communicate. The mature elder talks poetry or he doesn't talk!

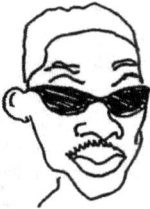

The mature human possesses supreme self-confidence and this sexy style *is* that man or woman. Due to panoramic vision he understands love when most complicated, terrifying, hilarious and true and he can love a woman at her worst: driven, obsessed, jealous or threatening. Younger men are always judging stereotypically (old-young, male-female, rich-poor) while older men have seen too many surprises for that. A woman is freer with the elder--as he ages he is more her model for his *panoramic vision*. The appreciation of true mature beauty comes with age for when free of blinding habits one can see (and communicate) "eternity". This was Einstein's greatest interest: what is eternity? Only through the elder can we even begin to grasp the sense of timeless space bringing this reality of God—joy! It's the master's toy—true perception, ever-changing and never deranging. Talks with the elder are a creative lift as through so much confusion he can sift. In youth we feel the rift (I was always miffed) but with age we see the gist—unless we are an ageist. For those who cling to sin to curb age-anxiety fall down to the cultural (non-natural) view of beauty which rejects themselves, more so with age (hardly the sage). But those who face the reality of nature become their own world's rage.

SEXY OLDER WOMEN

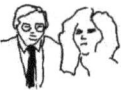

The best thing about the older man is his ability to appreciate the older woman. Can he? Belle aging in women is elegance, wholesomeness and sweetness together--the rare lady. The true lady is gentle worldliness, not seduction or feminism. The older man sees eternity in her--she represents it all in one ever-changing symbol: always-lovely, well-groomed, long-married, durable, reassuringly stable, home-and-heart devoted, responsible, respectable. She loves everyone in her charge. The man who loves this wife is the most revered and together they make the royal couple. A good example is Joanne Forsythe, an adored wife, called "my

107

lady" with reverence by a husband who adored her for what the wife could do, constantly providing settings where the world could see what he saw in her. These men are the best role models for floundering husbands, for their long marriages mellowed them out, making them honestly affectionate while their strong male presence was expanded. That's all any Queen ever wanted, or demanded. A faithful loving husband is the best man ever landed.

THE SELF-CONFIDENCE OF EXEMPLARS

These older men could have acted through sex stereotypes but they didn't want to for their charm increased by being more *themselves* as the seasons passed. Their victory over time was to *embrace* it for their character and *personality increase with age*. Self-confidence takes the prize as sex appeal grows from years of interaction. Those in the know see older as better—it's the difference between a rat and an Irish Setter. If men want to be authentically magnetic (sexy) they should heed the advice of this letter.

ELDER WRITERS

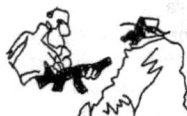

The same holds true in the arts: of those unmasking the young tarts or dirty old men breaking hearts. The older writer opinion leader is invisible—he's only the vessel through which inspiration comes. He is out of the way yet ever-present, a present from God, an exemplar and yet a paradox whom few know and many hate. Being above logic, gravity and age he is paralogic---known and controlled only by God who makes no sense to carnal man. Even he doesn't know why he writes what he does--he just does it and this is the highest possible path: giving up reasoning and acting from instinct made more automatic through the years as he transcends society. The older human is true (not cultural) wisdom, because he represents eternity and universal (not cultural) truths. With time his habits dissolve which maintain the ego—making him more humble, more transcendent and universal and more loved. What did his ego create when young? By the herd (and critics) he was shoved.

COASLESCENCE
Like an Underwater Observatory

ARTS OF PALEO FASTING

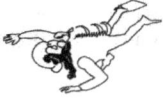

Aging is hard for women. Having received their worth from childbearing years past they may mourn this loss but then enter a new joyous phase of *coalescence*, a postmenopausal stage where everything learned to this point comes together at the summit. It's like an underwater observatory: This cues the fascinating phase of life-review with intense, lucid recall of sights, smells and feelings. Capturing these little gems is far more interesting than outer entertainment. These little "sparks" of recall may only bore others--like fasting, prayer, or dreams they should be enjoyed alone. If I were to recount these reviews to a friend I would miss the next jewel sparked in consciousness. All through history these postmenopausal single females ("crones") were rarely taken seriously or burned as witches (too psychic or they use herbs). But to the wise they are respected as loving harbingers of new life, health and wealth—an intuitive helper who's too busy to abide the intrusion of society. These single eccentrics live longest and are the most productive: now free they can give the most to an orphaned and lost world. The crone is the Biblical "eunuch" valued by God over the married woman--as the former loves God first, the latter loves spouse and world for the worst.

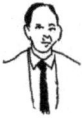

The *inability to handle intrusion* is a mark of genius and spirituality in the very private "cerebrotonic", or savant-autistic (socially separate wizard). Clever crones want only the company of God--for nothing else compares as each moment is so packed with fascination no human dare distract from this bliss. The married take orders from spouse and world, the single enjoy peace with God. Crones and singles: enjoy. The carefree crone is simply someone who no more puts up with puffed-up, prideful, pitiful personalities. That release few can ever know for it's knowing God instead. It's the absence of being filled with dread like the earlier social life she led. I love being married, but it's good to know with the inevitable.

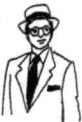

Crones have a detached capacity to love without need. Far from lonely they have a great life as people *instinctively flow in* for their uncanny advice. In contrast the fear of age becomes a no-exit trap called *avidya*, or ignorance, by the Hindus: a state of unawareness, fearful contraction and clinging that denies access to the future where all the glory lies. People who can't look ahead with great anticipation may back into the future--moving onward while clinging to what is gone forever. With this age-apprehension one sees only dark failures, broken plans, regrets/resentments, unresolved and ruptured relationships--the emotional "hot-spots" darkening the moment. Shutting off the future leaves nothing but physical decline. When old grudges arise you must think: "from this old thing I resign."

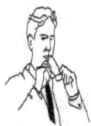

Resisting time while editing out age signs leads to depression or a blank psychic field like Alzheimer's Disease. When you reject the truth you are forced to accept a lie--that youth is superior and that aging is sadly inferior. Not so. Paradoxically, only conscious aging--accepting death--frees and releases our burden, for without shame or guilt the acceptance of death is the only thing releasing True Elder Beauty. Fear brings wrinkles, the joy of acceptance brings translucency of complexion and thrills (tingles). Laughter brings health and cheer makes one dear. To everyone who knows the clever caring crone she dries the tear and removes all fear for if you're going to heaven the future is blissfully clear.

THANATOS IS LIFE—FREE OF STRIFE

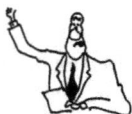

The denial of death is a safety valve in youth-"save life at any cost"--as threats trigger the fight-flight response with a flood of adrenaline. But this interferes with eldering when we just need to *contemplate* to feel the joyful insights of *thanatos*--in total calmness. Only by facing age as part of this mystical journey can we find wisdom and courage for in confronting death we gain a new orientation in life. Purged of myopic self-interest we awake to the splendors of the moment and little things: flowers, birds, puppies, friends--we can now serve others. Having been liberated from youth-obsession we become future-oriented—discounting the negative "old" image by showing the world our zest, joy, service and deep symbolic meaning to everything. I felt like I walked into a Maxfield Parrish painting or the wizard of oz. In every magical moment, what a feeling as everything learned before colors with perfect analysis (God's laws). Without being fear-led, I'm hitting the nail on the head. Now free of dread, I'm attracting the masses instead. I'm happy to help for I'm being led. That is mystical eldering—it's finally being *read*. Having faced death I'm ruddy with life (I'm red.)

HOMELIFE NO STRIFE

Holy heavenly home life is essential for happy eldering. Only in my own home am I'm protected from the ignorance right outside the door. Inside my cozy

ARTS OF PALEO FASTING

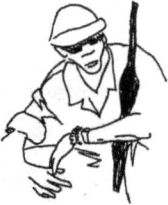

cabin encamped in cleverness and creative action I am free of the silly and mean in this godless era. Home life quiets ageist fears for if hooked to the herd one's dignity is smeared. Stay with your own—that's in your own domain, your home. That's the attraction of destiny like Rome. Free of panic, renewed energy pushes open the door to your happy "latter phase". I'm so happy I'm half-crazed. Look forward, you'll be amazed. But if part of the herd you'll be hazed, for the world's full of cruel idiots the Devil raised.

COMING TO TERMS WITH THE PAST

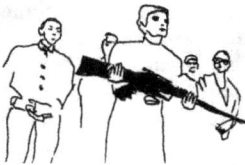

Coming to terms with the past was hard for me, taking decades to stop feeling ashamed and guilty. Every morning I'd wake-up either with a chip on my shoulder (more like a boulder) or extreme guilt (great tumult). It was facing death which dissolved the burden—for who cares now? Most of the judge-and-jury was dead so I thought: "no more of this dread!". I cannot describe what a relief this was, like moving from a concentration camp to a lovely fairy tale with me the star of Oz. This is the greatest thing about aging--we feel so light and joyous as the past dissolves and the future opens. It's so bright, I'm filled with might. But in order to enter this blissful inner sanctuary we must review the past in a healthy light--by recontextualizing our failures into successes (see it all in a new light), releasing resentments (now we're high as a kite), and reconnecting to unlived life we sacrificed on the way (would a midlife career change end the fight?)

LIFE REVIEW—"WHEW"

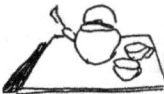

The main task of eldering is to reflect on the wealth of our past experiences. Once life review is set off we have a kaleidoscope of perceptions and revelations like bursts of exhilarated energy. These are lucid sights, sounds and smells that so enrich experience that both life review and enjoying the moment become intense explorations. Eldering is the time of the receptive mode and all the joys of relating to eternity: The phantasmagoria of our own rich history combined with sun-moon-stars. These powerful God-made forces were blocked out in the tunnel-vision of youth's pursuits. It is the flame of accepted mortality which opens this abundant life as we can now see the entire past differently just as the present--elemental reality of planets and angels--is transformed in our eyes. Our era of conquering and enduring cold love is now over so we can now see everything in a brand new light.   Now the pain is gone we can see the good in all while staying gentle like a fawn though walking tall.

ELDERS ESCAPE EARLY ESTIMATES

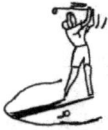

God says "my thoughts are not your thoughts." We thought we were right but now see we were wrong. We see how much betrayal and treachery were triggered by our own sins. We were blind to our own foibles which were clearly visible to others who reacted accordingly. In youth we jumped to conclusions, now re-examined in maturity. In youth we saw the world as for or against us--a view reinforced by hurtful betrayals conspicuous in mind. As age brings breadth these views are bashed as we see why they turned. Eldering is escape from the prison of early conclusions for the facts were there but our conclusions were wrong!

GOD TURNS ALL-BAD TO ALL-GOOD
Christ's Answer to the Hood

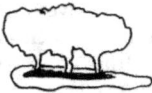

The self is still stuck in past pain where stunted experience cries to be healed--we've left home but the wounded child still weeps. Eldering sets the prisoners free: It is *inner repair* which releases us from jail—unresolved, we always fail. The past of strained relationships, sudden trauma, our own sins and incorrigible irritants forced us into peculiar adaptations. But now we get a sweet lesson: these negatives produced the real successes of maturity. Taking a new look we can say "yes" to the pearls the paltry (even perverted) past pains imparted for in all cases--no matter what occurred, God turns all-bad to all-good for those who love Him (all bad history becomes blurred). My biggest shames overcome, I can help misfits all over the world. Life review shows the true gains coming from loss: the realm beyond guilt-ridden anxiety reveals the hidden benefits in the sauce. As mature adults looking back we do reconstructive surgery on ourselves.   Free of the past and society--in synchrony with nature--we've become elves. Dusty dank memories we've put on the shelves. Instead we go deep inside--the domain into which every spiritual giant delves.

SIN BROUGHT HATE—THEY WERE IRATE

ARTS OF PALEO FASTING

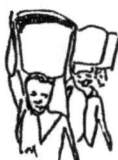

In eldering we see how sin removed our protection from foes as evil flowed in bringing us to lows. And all these years we blamed everybody else (even friends were seen as foes). Or we see how mere openness to evil elements put us in exile--from ourselves, God and His protections. All we ever had to do was just say NO to flesh and world--our people-tragedies were self-created. Having swallowed that bitter pill, we can now take total pleasure in the senses, free of all obsessive-compulsion. For true pleasure is non-compulsive, bringing no offenses.

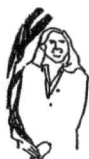

I was bitter over destiny but now feel grateful to be alive, having survived all the challenges just trying to survive. Are you riddled with resentment? Reframe your failures into success by giving testimony for life's severest teachers: list all the past foes and *invite them back mentall*y, thanking them for good coming from bad. This alchemy--making gold on aging resentments--converts resentment into gratitude, acceptance and peace. You'll be amazed at how it all fits—how they led to your divine best (in bits). The worst in life--the greatest losses of dignity--led to your crest. But it's final forgiveness which fills you with zest.

FORGIVENESS

Forgiveness reformats the templates driving us wild. Using the device of time-stretching we reach back to repair the hurts, broken promises, acts of betrayal and unhealed scars closing our hearts. The grudge keeps us in the dark--there is no creativity, energy or jubilance here as we become stark (just an angry bark). Forgiveness (embarrassingly) reveals our own role in the dysfunction and thus we face our shadow--the despised, rejected inner self who trips us up. Self-forgiveness for unconsciously creating the toxic situation unites and then releases the foe as friend for greater life and love. Did your arrogant, stubborn behavior create conflicts? Did the grasping nature of sin trigger cruel hatred in those closest? Daily forgiveness facilitates life harvesting and healing for hatred hampers immunity. (Were you not "sick" and "ugly" with unforgiveness?) Reject resentment or fail and die. Forgive, take the throne, and prolong your life or bye-bye.

Now, because you faced death and reframed your history
you've extended your life accordingly.

WORRY

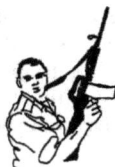

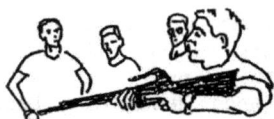

Fear gets you away from danger but worry is a sin of mental attitude. It's not just concern when things don't go right but failure to understand God's provision and promises. It's failure to "cast our care upon Him." Without faith we enter soul-torment or anxiety—a painful state of "undue concern" or more accurately utter torment from the lower side of hell. Worry shocks the body like a bludgeon. Aren't you sick of this dungeon? Through muck and mud you've been trudgin'. I'd rather go light—there's only one way to float like a kite. That means to not take that first bite of worry, the Devil's spite. It's a very old story preventing Victory, but no more once worry's out of the armory. The only way to be happy and worry-free is to trust God for all things. Worry is a projection of sin and it destroyed your kin. With repentance people become carefree—that's the only way to be, as God our only protector takes care of our entire destiny. For He had it all planned beforehand—it's all worked out as far as you can see.

WORRY ANTICIPATES THE WORST
Maturity is Stability

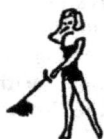

God wants us to be happy—as His kids we come first. If worry the mind-enemy fills us with God-thirst, it can be beneficial. But usually it becomes a painful apprehension of misfortune, trouble or uncertainty. It makes us restless, agitated and painfully confused. Wouldn't you rather be enthused? When finally free, by everything (even housework) you'll be amused, but worry destroys all so it needs to be loosed. For sooner or later the fearful are bruised. Why go through all that when you could have cruised? When all you had to do was pray: With God's miraculous light be infused, for worry destroys the body especially if boozed. As sin caused fear and dependency, by others you are used, and from low self-esteem you're sorely abused as you cave-in when being accused. On the subject of worry I bemused: "shouldn't this be diffused?" After I let it go my dear Father excused. Due to fear-sin, the devil's crowd (whom you call in fear) mis-use. I stopped my worry after God's words to me I perused: "This mind trap you'll now refuse. Now we can work--no more you being cast off unused."

WORRY DESTROYS SOUL & BODY
Mis-Applied Energy to Tangents

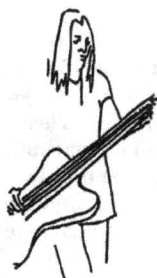

Worry misdirects us into useless tangents seeking glory and it's not cute after forty. If unchecked worry becomes mental illness. First you're warned through worry itself—if it goes on beyond the initial shock of change, it's a bad sign. Then it manifests physically as it shocks the body like a knife. Defenses down, we become a clown. We get ill from hysteria—even getting malaria. Everyone has certain areas in which they are prone to worry, encouraging others in the same. Watch who your influences are—it's them you must tame. People can always find something about which to worry so cut loose nosy meddlers (those worry-peddlers). For even from kin it's still a sin. Learn to ride with the flow—God can turn this aggravation into dough (for you, because you're in the know). So accept the new circumstances although I know it can't be easy—whirlwind changes like broken borders (sudden surroundings by strangers) can really make us wheezy.

WORRY LEADS TO SIN & MORE WORRY

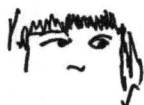

It's worry vs. Victory. Worry causes backsliding which automatically creates more worry. Yes that worry comes from sin: You slip, you burn, your heart will churn so stop the rut and learn or these thought-demons you'll never spurn. Without this life-blight you're ready to earn. I don't want to be stern but you must make a turn so new life and bounty can fill your urn. Look to the vistas and think of eternity, the good life for which you yearn. That height of joy you must *earn* (then you can sequester yourself from crowds and chaos—turning inward or burn). To mental torture say "adjourn." Give up all concern and just laugh for the angels return. It's like a fragrant fern but while in sin there are accidents and more earthly concern. Now make that turn—enontiodromia will turn it all around and bring back more: double for your trouble, like a big tax return.

WORRY FROM GUILT

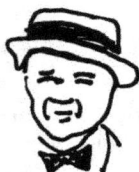

Worry is sin so God commands us to stop worrying and to fret not evil doers. You must repent to be free of this stinging bee warping the whole family tree. Believe me--I paid a terrible fee and it's no way to be. Obey God's decree: from this sin you must flee as it shows you don't trust Him, see? I mean gee don't you want your childhood glee? Look to God for only He is the key. Banish your ego just sit at his knee for without Him you've the power of a flea. The herd doesn't help though you feel power in "we" (they seem to agree then on you they pee, Oui?) There's no strength in numbers (it's all debris) but join the divine--it's like a spending spree. So you have a degree? You're still as small as a pea. Look at me--I was so bourgeoisie until from worry I became an absentee, as to all fearful thoughts I decided to disagree. Just trust God and do your own work for I guarantee that starts a jubilee (don't worry and life's a potpourri). If you can turn your worry into creativity, you'll write as well as Williams, Tennessee. To a extreme degree please remember my plea: worry's as deep as the sea. That endless CD is not the Marquis who wins the battle for the mind--do you see? Then over all problems you'll skate/ski.

CRUTCH NEVER WORKS--IT JUST ERKS
To Become Great Sometimes We First Grate

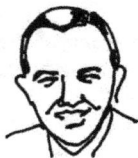

For some people, in order to be very great they have to first get very bad, in preparation for conversion to the opposite. It's the same intense energy creating both extremes, and it's our losses of dignity that teach us more than anything else. Did you get soused or become a louse? Don't worry as inversion to the opposite builds your glory house. That's the cross you had to bear (becoming bad in the world's glare) but understanding enantiodromia can remove the worry-scare (it will now erase and you'll be without care). For worry doesn't solve problems it only blinds us to the answers. One must control emotions to see clearly, as they distort reality. The champions control the most distorting, warping emotion of all—worry. For anxiety creates tension and tension erodes joy and when joy is gone victory is lost, faith is weakened and spontaneity is destroyed. The spirit falls ill. How can God use us if we've lost our joy? I like to think this way: in fifty or a hundred years it'll all be gone—in oblivion, it won't annoy. As the song says "May your dreams come true, there's no need to cry for I will be with you. Together we'll find a way, so trust in Me girl [boy]."

RECAP

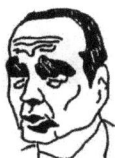

Worry makes one ugly and aged: it distracts from the goodness of God. Your Father desires you be happy every moment, but sin punishes with worry. And God's blessing for repentance is: freedom from worry. The weary warping worn-out sin of worry is strictly forbidden yet in prayer and fasting you can ask God for anything and He will answer you. It's True especially for sinners too.

P.S.

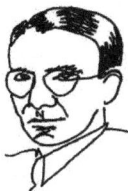

To not worry don't give yourself something to worry about from sin or bad association. Have no contact for then it's *influence*, then *conquest*. I felt as though I lived in a sea of sharks. It was hard to know who to trust. The new age counterfeit was everywhere justifying everything. I finally saw how to live: carve out my own domain and destiny and just stay there. Knowing its a sea of sharks I would just skillfully navigate around the Jim Dandy's, charity candies and shifty-called-"Saintly" Sandy's. My failing was not knowing they were sharks then stupidly going out to play with them. Yes it's always a case of a wolf in sheep's clothing: Of course the sharks are going to live through a healthy, saintly, philanthropic, animal and child loving, evil-hating and God-loving "image"—that's their line of scrimmage. To banish worry I learned to "trust no man" especially those spouting spiffy new age holier-than-thou false fronts. Never forget: skillfully navigate--every single moment you must skillfully navigate through the lushes and losers living (influencing) and so-called "loving" through images and symbols. If we can't see through the mirage there's a call from the subconscious and justified worry takes over. So now be silent, coy, mysterious and don't lose your cover. Just stay silent, do your work and win all because you said "worry move over."

ARTS OF PALEO FASTING

OLD SONGS SAID IT BEST

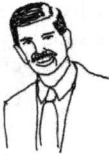

Forget your troubles and just get happy. Better chase all your cares away... get ready for the judgment day... The sun is shining so get happy. The Lord is waiting to take your hand, we're going to the promised land. We're heading across the river: Wash your sins away in the tide for it's all so peaceful on the other side.

Take a mental vacation, you must! How can God in-fill if you're stuck in some groove or trackin' the public?

LONELINESS

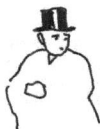

How well I know the feeling. The pitiful fear in
the gut. Why is it always that rut? We feed so
that feeling will cut.

ALONE, GENIUS COMES OUT

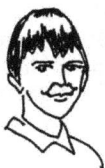

Being alone does not mean lonely because solitude is restorative--
it's the only way for certain talents to erupt and alight. After
being alone genius is filled with might: no more spite, now he's
brilliant with light. You'll see I'm right if you try it without getting
tight—for the problems of the hypersensitive are reactive to
misjudgment. Solitude develops true self-confidence to heal and
rebuild (see this and your lifelong fight ends by tonight).

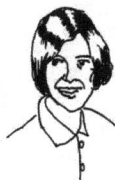

On my Inner Journey there were times I felt I would lose my mind
with loneliness, so I'd take steps to be with people or to
"join". These stop-gaps were always pit-falls for I'd always
draw back into privacy with gratitude—oh my sweet solitude! I
wasn't ready to come back freshly endowed with new powers for
the necessary life-phase of being happy alone was still
incomplete. We molt when we molt, a chicken lays an egg when
it's supposed to—and that's that. Those times of social hunger just indicate
you still need solitude. When I finally realized this I felt so free (I cooed).

SOLITUDE'S A CERTAIN SOLACE

The Bible shows how special singleness and solitude is, for singles have a
unique ability to focus completely on spiritual things. Jesus' example showed

119

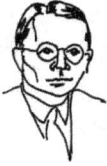

solitude as a time for energizing meditation as he retreated to lonely places to pray and strengthen himself to deal with the crowds. Solitude is an affirming, energizing, happily divine time. And if you can learn to tolerate it you'll soon enjoy it with gratitude, for it gives you such latitude! Having stretched your psychic survival skills when alone you'll be socially stronger (not so willing to slide) when popularity comes back.

CONTRARY TO POP OPINION

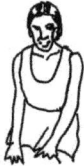

If lonely, filling yourself with people, things and demands will never bring contentment for it's only in solitude and reflection that the True Self is found. Alone we can be who we really are—who God called us to be and thus it should be the best time of our lives. Revel in it for you'll lose it soon enough, for if you can garnish all its benefits you may never have it again. Whenever lonely say that to yourself: "sadly I may never have this special time again." Reverse what you think—it's depression you'll cheat. Soon you'll heal all whom you meet for you're pretty and sweet: After being solo everything's on easy street, so enjoy this necessary retreat.

PANACEAS FOR PRIVACY "PAIN"
It's Just a Misconception—Again

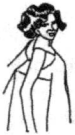

Here are some suggestions to deal with the terrible feeling of loneliness, a pandemic feeling as most families and marriages break up. The first lesson is self-gentleness: treat yourself like a pup. Learn how to be alone for the end is the mountaintop. Endure this temporary retreat for if you can see the whole picture your heart won't erupt (it's finding your True Self, so don't stop).

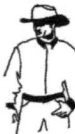

It's easy to buy Hollywood's trip that "romance" fixes that feeling— not true. Loneliness indicates we've lost our way—our connection to our spirit, heart and destiny. Know God puts us in solitude to strengthen and fine-tune our reflections about life self and others. Though it hurts temporarily it's the only way to release those talents of the true self bringing us to perfect success. Knowing that, we can just sit back and watch the whole fantastic show which is triggered by solitude—no people, just pets (walks with dog, talks with God).

ARTS OF PALEO FASTING

WE MAKE IT WORSE

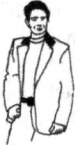

It's hard offsetting the constant cultural messages since childhood that we're incomplete unless attached and that solitude is to be avoided. Due to the suspicious harassments as to why we "haven't found the right one" we feel incomplete—a mistaken identity. Don't take this on (it's a cultural con) for it'll encumber you a ton. Just seek the sun and you will have won (it means mon).

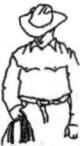

As you can now see loneliness is made more intense by what you tell yourself it means. Especially youth is susceptible to these misconceptions: that it's a sign of weakness, immaturity, inferiority, personality defect or that they are the only one feeling it. If you bought this you slipped into problems of self-assertion, social risk-taking, enjoyment at parties, responsiveness to others. You're cynical, mistrusting and unable to self-disclose. You've begun blaming/judging, expecting rejection and getting even more critical, depressed, angry, afraid and misunderstood--self-pity has set in. What unnecessary traps. Don't ever start this false path for this mis-labeled loneliness is perpetuated through discouragement-in-isolation. Or the opposite occurs: becoming involved too fast without evaluating the consequences create sick (unsatisfying) relationships or worse: over-commitment to a bad faith relationship that destroys decades. If only you'd have seen solitude in a spiritual light this would never have happened.

We were in our own sight grasshoppers and
so we appeared to them. Numbers 13: 33

WE ALL FEEL LONELY

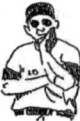

Loneliness is a common experience, so conquering it puts one far ahead of the game (to be happy even with the rain). What one learns after a painful era of loneliness is that *people really don't care* but God does and He's always there. If we can be satisfied with Him he gives us total creative fun all day (social hunger will never pay that way). One-quarter of all Americans feel painful loneliness every few weeks and youth feel it even more. It is neither permanent or bad, just an indicator of imagined unmet needs making us sad.

ARTS OF PALEO FASTING

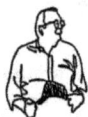

To end that desolate lonely feeling just keep telling yourself (1) it's necessary for your ultimate success (2) it's temporary—it won't last forever (3) it's building character (4) it's something for you to return to in mind when things go wrong— your "wonderful vacation in privacy" (5) it's evoking your True Genius. Get it? You need it so you can lead the flock, so don't look back look ahead (forget the clock). So this wonderful time don't mock for you're about to shoot to a new plane on which you'll be locked. I really loved these twenty years (I rocked).

IT'S ONLY TEMPORARY

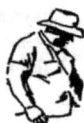

OK so solitude may only be temporary. Use it to get to know your soon-to-be-famous self. Become herd-independent to take care of your own emotional needs without the crutch of using others to fulfill them. Stop being a user. If you do this you'll be way ahead of the human race who are stuck in ruts--sick systems and cycles keeping them down as clown (hardly renown). Champs must seclude not only to avoid the lewd and the rude but also for success—to make a new dent that changes the race forever. Are you yet that clever? Then in that pursuit revel in this leisure, this special time of silent glory without measure (it's a fine treasure).

ENJOY THYSELF

The jail-guards are gone, so use this time to enjoy yourself (rather than just existing) until you're again with others. Avoid merely vegetating—deal with your situation actively for you are learning such an important lesson: how to entertain yourself and find your true interests and hobbies. Be a hobby-horse like the smart adolescent (this time you won't be derailed by hormones kicking in). You can re-achieve the hobbyhorse happiness by cultivating this much higher state. It's hardly third-rate or coming-late (you're missing nothing—forget getting a "mate"). For in silence its finally harvest time, a gold-mine. Recognize that there are so many creative and enjoyable ways to use your time alone. Use your unique interests to fill your time as an ex-clone.

RECAP—IT'S YOUR MAP

ARTS OF PALEO FASTING

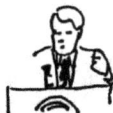

Soon you'll be broadcasting to the masses of asses, so don't ever define yourself as a lonely person. If you open up to destiny and pursue your fasting ideas you are never lonely nor bored. No matter how bad or sad loneliness disappears as you focus on current needs to make your life better--right at this moment on this day. Are you ready to receive the ray? Love eternity in stars, moon, sun today and you'll always be OK come what may.

P.S.

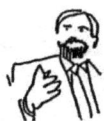

There are no victories without battles. Conquer this problem to fight the good fight. It means taking a fasting (on people, habits or food) flight. Enjoy thyself--that's being a knight. Get into your own unique destiny and see this as a temporary bullet to bite. It's pure joy you'll be feeling today and tonight.

PALEO POWER AND OBLIGATE CARNIVORES

I'm an Obligate Carnivore. Carnivores eat fruit and leaves. It's a matter of proportion, which varies.

Carnivores eat fruit and leaves. Even if a little lemon on their fish, it's fruit and I love yogurt with berries.

When I finally ate cheese after decades of rabbit food my whole world opened up in a colorful phantasmagoria.

Fauna is not a dirty thing but what we're supposed to eat. I may not like it either but truthfully I sure feel great.

I'm satisfied from next to nothing cuz it's the right thing: Morning is fauna and milk, later 2 grapes/I'm full.

The onslaught from ex-veganism is ruthless and vicious so you must now man-up to enjoy the delicious.

It's funny how everything is opposite: Meat-eaters have stable moods/are peaceful, not the rabbit-fooders.

I noticed meat-eating men looked very handsome like the carnivorous actors from way back when.

It's totally enjoyable switching from meat to fruit and back again. They are a perfect balance to maintain.

Marinate your meats with fruits like berries. It's meat and fruits that go together and rabbits eat the veggies.

Two grapes and I was full, satisfied. You don't have to eat truckloads like they say, just balance/even pies.

Balance: Eat fruit then balance with meat. Fast, then balance again and it's all instructed by your system.

ARTS OF PALEO FASTING

Many vegans are so deficient they dream of pot roast every night. A very dangerous thing/a blight.

MacDougal reasons: since all continents exist on starch it must be right. That's typical liberal science, hah.

In the fifties when people were handsome and pretty this woulda been a no-brainer: meat on the platter.

Now they make concoctions to replace meat and it's sickening, we won't even touch our plate.

Green powders stuck in liver: When ex-vegans take colonics to rid the past it's a a green snake they eject.

The future will laugh at this era when people bought pills, powders and potions and we all spent a fortune.

I'm so enjoying my yogurt raw-milk with coconut and two mango chunks, I'm high as a kite, fully stoked.

Don't discuss your diet cuz they all come down on you for it since there's always two sides so forget it.

Every plant and animal has self-defense--veggies don't wanna be eaten! That's why I get sick and hate em.

Fruits are ok but I prefer FATS. Animal fat (fauna) keeps my brain in tune, high energy, focus and gladness.

To think I tried to get the fat from avocado or nuts! How useless, I go right to the source of confusion.

Go ahead and stay on plant diet while I live life to it's fullest and am what I am cuz I eat what God gave us.

Gave my dogs raw beef yesterday--they ate it up so happily, now I see why they won't eat cooked meat.

ARTS OF PALEO FASTING

Put one pineapple chunk in my raw milk shake with yogurt. There, I had my fruit and I'm better for it.

Carnivores eat fruit and leaves. It's a matter of proportion which varies but right now via meat I'm sweet.

Keep veggies for rabbits cuz for humans they're filled with anti-nutrients--what a laugh since the 60's.

In the Old West they went to town once a month to get butter, bacon and coffee.

It used to be the roast was the main dish but now if you bring it you're seen as a murdering creep/accomplice.

All wrinkles leave body suddenly since it's same bloodstream running thru every cell/thank you daddy.

What is a feast? Something magnificent which allows you to fast 2-3 days afterwards at least.

After learning all about diets you ultimately have to be your own guru and then shut up about it.

With animal foods/no starch or sugar I experienced a Maxfield Parrish reality of castles and fairytales.

Animal foods diet means daily fasting cuz the satiety is implied: how lil' ladies stayed skinny in the fifties.

Ex-vegans attacked by vegans the same way liberals attack anyone who escapes their grip, how sick.

After resuming meat after decades: everything worked perfectly and that horrible dry skin went away.

Durianrider and Freelee reeled me back so many times, they're good salesmen of veganism I'll say that.

It was always the animal cruelty issue that made me drop new heath to truckle back in and avoid the feud.

ARTS OF PALEO FASTING

After meat: Wow! So THIS is how I'm supposed to feel--the way I did as a kid, before the shovedown pill.

It was beautiful people of the 50's-60's and it was stolen from them with margarine/lowfat doctrine.

I thought: Wow! So this is how I'm supposed to feel--the way I did as a kid, before the shovedown pill.

The beautiful people of the 50's-60's and it was stolen from them with margarine and lowfat doctrine.

It was always the animal cruelty issue that made me drop new heath to truckle back in and avoid the feud.

Low fat vegan dogma (shove down) hurt dogs too. They were deprived of table leavings/delicious food.

It's a food paradox: fruit makes ya bitchy as hell and meat makes you (again) a sweet little boy or girl.

When fat melted off and I got my synapses back, Wow: electricity running thru cholesterol is perfect.

I often switch from lowcarb to paleo all cuz I wanna eat fruit.

On vegetable oils like olive I had belly fat but when I substituted with animal fat it ALL went away.

Ate a pear and thought I'd die for a day. Gut ache: meat digests sooo smoothly and fiber is self-hate.

This comes from the severe digestive disorders resulting from veganism which has never occurred on earth.

Broccoli isn't even a real vegetable and many veggies poison eaters for protection/avoid em man.

Everything comes down to synapses and all wiring is insulated in fat which means lowfat diets = insanity.

ARTS OF PALEO FASTING

I was insane for decades from the lack of animal fat. Avocados didn't do it, olive oil nothing to it.

The irrational fear of meat--did you have it as a kid? No, we took it all for granted then, it was IT.

I felt like crap with all that fiber in the gut. With meat I'm so stable/smooth/sleek with high energy/strut.

Insulation for all wiring in us is cholesterol and that's the very thing they told us to avoid? Incredible

I don't like it any more than you do but I gotta do it to survive cuz, I'm sick with fiber, starch, sugar/no jive.

Ex-vegan carnivores eat meat and organs raw. Sorry I can't do that for it's enough just to eat it at all.

Lowfat = Weak control over actions/words as autonomisms (uprushes from the unconscious) occurred.

Finally, we don't have to fear vegan's reactions to our new direction pursuing wellness despite the angry.

I wasn't myself and could never be myself cuz that's based on animal fat which I cut out, just like that.

Eating meat even has to do with family bonding. They meet to eat, very important and warmin'

Anti-nutrients: That's what veggies have and I'm thinking of my uncle who refused em/only ate bread.

Since I gave up fiber I feel so much better. The gut unblocked from matter made me visibly fitter.

If you can't eat meat or non-fruit find one protein you can, regain your immunity then you can eat it all.

Haven't tried raw eggs yet but promise I'll get to it.

ARTS OF PALEO FASTING

Vegans are part of liberal cabal as well as NWO. Those who don't get sucked in maintain health in gold.

Even a little fiber and I have a truck in my gut. Obligate carnivores are fit/flat with all belly fat out.

They portray the anti-nutrients in plants and even soy as "healthy". They always do that and thus we die.

Over 80% of vegans/vegetarians go back to eating meat. Why, if it's so great and perfect for the peeps?

Bill Gates supports depopulation--and fake meat. Hmmm

Fake meat, NWO veganism = zombie apocalypse. Heck, can't you see it in their eyes as we speak?

Though it looks like a healthy trend veganism is actually Satanic. Hitler did it, heavy metal bands do it.

Hollywood is very into it, you hear about it everywhere. NWO brainwash, like Ellen eats her carrots.

I will not be surprised when all the liberal (FALSE) churches go vegan. Even now church sites are joining in.

Very prevalent now: Churches giving diet advice and vegan is in. They see it as holy/more virtue signalin'

Churches will be serving fake meats at their potlucks and no one would think of bringing a pot roast.

Used to be the guest bringing the beef roast was a real hero but not he'd be embarrassed to.

Ex-vegans all lost their teeth and now eat nothing but meat. They can't digest the rest/made em effete.

ARTS OF PALEO FASTING

Just as the water reflects the stars and the moon, the body reflects the mind and soul. Rumi quotes

The Walmart pie said "freshness guaranteed" as it stood fresh on the shelf for one year/don't believe.

When you eat, eat the most calorically dense possible--not rabbit food. Cowboy Levoy Finicum

My interest in daily fasting is not anorexia but a spiritual calling. Like some are called to celibacy, it's my thing.

With the wrong premise people lose their intelligence and they'll all see it when things don't add up.

ROAST at 375 for 3 hours: Cut tomatoes tossed with olive oil, salt, pepper and lotsa garlic--enjoy it.

Vegans say "no oil" but that's bull if you're in for the long haul. Potato chips: sliced/ S&P/olive oil, broil.

I learned at 15 I didn't have normal digestive apparatus with only one possible digestive burn a day.

I just wanna appreciate this day, a Saturday. I haven't eaten yet, why spoil it-- not hungry just wanna think.

Vegans are like all SJW's--rude and cruel as they hammer in the speel of the cool tyrannizing over you.

Restore old paths and 18" waists.

Lberal (vegan) persecution for eating meat is so violent and opprobrious most can't recover their health.

Many gurus of raw veganism admit to eating cooked food, ice cream or animal products--yet are selling this.

As a vegan I made poor decisions making me sicker then seeking of superfoods and snake oil potions etc.

ARTS OF PALEO FASTING

Vegans also promote vasectomies--stripping you of a future family and that is a cruel horrible tragedy.

And to think family complained of "hunger for something" and instead of giving em meat I gave em a seed.

I experimented with Daily Fasting *Eating Anything* for years to prove a point but now I want what's right.

Dogs are so happy with pot roast aromas going thru the house. They too see veganism as ridiculous.

Happy cute meat-eating kid. Met a man who called me unkind so I went vegan and lost health and mind.

Twenty years: acid burn as vegan. Thought I had esophageal cancer hon' but as an ex-vegan pain is gone.

As vegan I was so dizzy I often had to sit down. I lost immunity, every chemical affected me, frown.

Losing teeth, often angry, aging early and dry skin: that's the vegan and I'm sorry to pop your vision.

It's not ugly aging is from not eating meat. It's living on non-nutritive starches and sweet fruits/effete.

Vegan trip was part of liberalism and the globalist's plan to bring us down. Deficiencies of effete, overrun.

Proclamation: Forcing vegan dogma on cats and dogs is cruel and wrong!

The cruelty thing took over minds and we saw meat-eaters as evil and meat itself as dirty/despicable.

Vegans look great at first but as reserves are depleted and deficiencies rear up they fail to thrive/I lived it.

The vegan doctors had no credentials they just believe the credo, a mouthful.

ARTS OF PALEO FASTING

Like a giant conspiracy: Lure us to accept dogma making us sick so we buy your snake oil tricks.

No bigger clash: traditional meat eating family with a new vegan justice warrior looking like a horror.

When I went vegan at 22 I instantly developed an eating disorder but couldn't see it like Karen Carpenter.

Give em what they want/are hungry for: meat. Nothing else satisfies, seems nutritious or doesn't exist.

Why are patients given plant-based diet? To keep em in the system so there's no recovery to fight it.

Wanting meat so bad but not able to go against orthorexic dogma inside. Extremely dangerous/I tried it.

I would not eat the dirty thing--meat. The cruelty. So for years--decades--I continued but I'm back.

I feel so much better three days into the paleo-fast. Wow, wow, wow after years of hazy fatigue in the past.

Stop forcing your poor dogs and even cats to eat cauliflower you cruel creepy vegan monsters.

I hate to say it, I really do: but all the basic nutrients are in the meat not the plants and I'm sorry for you.

After years of confusion I'm filled with energy as an obligate carnivore which means fasting more.

Meat: After years of 10-banana smoothies etc. I have clarity/energy and what a lesson for America.

Ladies were beautiful/gents handsome but then in came low fat dogma and they became ugly/dumb.

ARTS OF PALEO FASTING

All were thin/good-looking but then TV ads said "no butter--just margarine" and we all succumbed.

To see an entire culture go from beauty and brains to dumb squares in pain is so telling/instructive, just sayin'

Many scientists knew it too: the way to bring down the west was to make em sick as hell and depressed.

Low-fat vegan so messed up my health now all I can eat is meat/zero-carb which reversed defeat.

Ruined metabolism thru lowfat vegan means you're now an obligate carnivore/ageless star.

The obligate carnivore sees disappearance of wrinkles, dry skin, baseless fears or nothing happenin'

Angelina Jolie--a world beauty--has bacon and eggs every morning then nothing, you see?

As a tired vegan I got addicted to caffein pills and ruined my health even more. Now not--energy galore!

Vegans are lousy workers. Being brain fogged/fuzzy they start to take superfoods and powders.

Powders, pills and potions don't work. They stay in the liver, a big slimy green ball making tiredness worse.

After losing my teeth from fruit-only diet I was still so utopian-brainfogged I argued with the dentist.

A happy meat eater as a teen, when I switched to vegan it was the worst eating disorder ever seen.

You take away a person's sustenance--the thing making him human and his True Self--and it's hell.

ARTS OF PALEO FASTING

What I went through for decades of mental illness and skinny fat unfitness was one for the Guinness.

What I went thru with the inability to handle people, the lack of boundaries and assertion against invaders/evil.

Just like an alcoholic goes to lowlife. it was the same with lost destiny from rejecting what I needed for life.

You can't develop musculature on anything but meat. Those vegan body builders are a scam, believe me.

Genius and saints are pure, kind to animals but that doesn't mean they are vegan--that's new age/false.

Switch from lowcarb to paleo when you wanna eat fruit.

Forget avocado, coconut, olive oil--it doesn't work for dry skin. Use butter baby, the real thin'

While writing of cornucopia I had no sense of it cuz I wasn't eating meat--it was illusion: child's view of utopia.

On the first meat day my whole life opened up and it was true cornucopia, vivid perception, lucid recall.

Here I was, an obligate carnivore due to low immunity and I removed my only lifeline due to virtue signaling.

Here I was, a sweet meateating child with huge potential who bought the trip that veganism was essential.

I became a ovo-lacto-rasta vegetarian but I'm afraid that wasn't enough. It's in the red meat, liver and blood.

The very things we needed to be handsome blueprints of humans and they said drop this dangerous vermin.

A pig is not like a rat--don't listen to that.

ARTS OF PALEO FASTING

Stop forcing your poor dogs and even cats to eat cauliflower you cruel creepy vegan monsters.

The whole point of the meat is I don't have to eat again, see? But it's where the minerals are they tell me.

Low fat vegan dogma (shove down) hurt dogs too. They were deprived of table leavings/delicious food.

It's a food paradox: fruit makes ya bitchy as hell and meat makes you (again) a sweet little boy or girl.

When fat melted off and I got my synapses back, wow: electricity running thru cholesterol is perfect.

P.S. Carnivores also eat fruit. That's when you go from lowcarb to paleo.

As you get clear from right foods you realize how many have victimized you in your lowered state--whew!

A. SELFHOOD OBSTRUCTIONS

Early rejection explains the insane drive for greatness and the survival panic leading to suicide.

Devil holds us back through remorse. Trigger-memories: anchors holding us down to the bad past.

Significance comes from identity of being a child of God and that gives you a purpose/not seen as odd.

The world imposes it's BS then weak friends get sucked in/create a mess and then they're high maintenance.

They don't want you to succeed. That needs to be focused on and wondered about, don't you agree?

To succeed keep auditing your network for signs of friendship vs. frenemyshit. Are they even interested?

Do they create contention/division, are they predators of the heart, do they not want you to succeed?

Audit Network: Do they hold you to the past and not want you to advance to your destiny and future?

Friendship is very rare/must be prized and held onto until you die. Problem is: world comes in, then bye bye.

The time is late, you've achieve something so great so now audit your network lest demons change your fate.

Do they want you to succeed? Or are they acting like a rudder bogging you down into the gutter?

Told to get along with her 1000 cousins of course she's validating sin in this era of porn and cruisin'.

It takes a long time to become young. Picasso

It wasn't just that. Things had been brewing under the surface and I just chose that event to wrap it up.

You got to cut em loose or you'll stay nothing, a caboose. They're not up to your par so fire em or lose.

Prosperity cannot be proof of God's favor since it's what Satan promises for those worshipping him.

All sins are attempts to fill voids. It's like a huge suction cup and in comes horrible things to avoid.

Imaginary evil is romantic and varied but real evil is monotonous, gloomy, barren and extremely boring.

Imaginary good is boring but real good always new, marvelous, relieving and intoxicating. S. Weil

Real good is the BEST--but kids don't see that, being sold a bunch of lies. Be good genius and open eyes.

ARTS OF PALEO FASTING

You need a hobby or a true cause. not this weird extreme crap, it's deeply evil on the way to hell.

It was the devil you hated, not me. In weakness I bent and he overtook the vessel in my life's tragedy.

Driven by identity-panic cuz if I didn't work I wouldn't survive it: that's the history of all who made it.

Why bring up age? It's just abuse. I move and feel like I'm fifteen and work every waking minute too.

After you reject/fire the creep take a day to convalescence cuz you've felt damage with his mess.

Forgive: leave psychic space completely OPEN so God can fill it with ceaseless miracles one after another!

But the time is up for those who are corrupt.

I had to go through life in two stages: learning thru hurting (Ph.D. in the Streets) *then* success/reaping.

Stop cowering/sinking in your swill. These are all past tapes when you were overcoming and learning still.

The sinner should say: "I just want my intended life back."

It's horrifying what I'm finding out about em so more and more I'm succumbin' to being in my own cocoon.

Be smart you cute one you, don't read your reviews.

It's the end of a long haul, a monumental achievement so now go slow, be deliberate, take it easy.

Don't fret you didn't follow your plan cuz it's all about God's plan, man! And that's what you've been doin'

ARTS OF PALEO FASTING

Just because they find you unworthy of their attention you desperately want their attention more, amen?

Don't resent past tyrants just see the system that brought it on: you were sick, addicted, negligent, down.

I'm off at noon, the Lord said He wanted receptivity--a switch from the tunnel vision of work obsession.

Feel as though I'll never get over it: Tyrants over me and kids invading me and I couldn't stand up to it.

It built certain muscles in me: constantly having to battle to get privacy, it ordered my life, you see.

The Lord wanted me solo so he put me thru people hell until I learned: lock the gate/end psychic smell.

How to complete a project: Lay out the frame, fill in the dots.

As the body recedes in old age the brain expands--imagine that.

Because I am maximally receptive the dark night of the soul was horrible, reading thoughts/no miracles.

I'm done, the ten world changing blockbusters are ready for ebook distribution or paperbacks if you choose.

Young love is about passion old love about accommodation--protecting the other's solitude in sun.

You're done with your work now it's just final touches, massage into perfection, deal with markets.

Now done, turn your attention to another world. Release tunnel vision as you open up/avoid the lure.

I'm done with my work, it's locked into place. Now talking about the work: how man is disgraced.

ARTS OF PALEO FASTING

Collaboration isn't always the key to success. More often they drag you down and the design's a mess.

He can't see, he doesn't remember me but he still loves Thee.

A rising tide rises all ships--I'll reward those helping. That's not me bragging I feel what's happening.

It's the complex human race in it's weird intricacies and devices to maintain homeostasis making us nuts.

Free willers scare me—they don't know the wonderful destiny God designed for free.

They don't search for the predestined groove we have with repentance, see?

Style to the end. Either you have it or you don't, friends

If you're an unread author what good are you?

This poetry came from deep emotions as I recall the lessons/never forget em.

Until it goes into production there are corrections! Now's not the time for complacency--focus!

Ten books and a billion details and it's all going into production and it's chaos and I love this.

To sell books ya gotta have the fame and you get that by goin' against the grain.

To feel really good look how far you've come. You're not done yet but man have you been accomplishin'.

3/4 there--gonna go real slow to the finish line to make sure I didn't forget something/got the weekend.

Gonna party while I finish all weekend. Lookin' forward to the new life which will be opposite, yes ma'am.

ARTS OF PALEO FASTING

You're 99.99% done but don't rush the finish, hon'! Handle like a crate of eggs, take the whole weekend.

Key to a masterpiece is *patience*. Never rush it just savor ride into completion and world success.

Hats off to my tech guy adapting to my extreme Harriet Craig attention to detail in this masterpiece.

You have reached a point in completion where even you can't muck it up.

You're done, hon'. It's just a matter of filling in the dots a bit more so today just party on/celebration

Oh come on, even he doesn't have all the answers. Stop this people worship and get back to nature.

Oh come on, even I don't have all the answers. Don't worship me or anyone else sir.

Your time has come.

I'm done, my time has come and now we'll have fun after a long haul of decades overcoming dung.

She said I had delusions of grandeur. Please Lord, show her.

It took many decades but much of that was just suffering, learning and overcoming not writing.

Abnormal Psychology or Interactional Pathology (Systems Theory)?

Once planting a seed instead of fearing "it" won't happen, get ready--for God said He would bless it, see?

I'm not gonna discuss my plans with you, why jinx em? You don't know what it is/what it took dumb dumb.

The fastest way to ruin your life is discuss it with anyone so refuse to answer their insinuating questions!

ARTS OF PALEO FASTING

You don't know anything about my life, what I do or what it's taken so shut fruitless questions/bye.

If someone has the truth they say it simply and if they don't they blab on falsely.

It's surival panic for a comic to engage people, coming from a neglectful mother and he'll do anything for it.

When you don't have a loving connection with the mother it's almost impossible to be disliked later.

Due to early rejection writers want world's approval 1000% and since that can't happen, die of alcoholism.

Steeped in resentments of dead long ago I am overwhelmed with survival panic fearing books unsold.

We're not at the end but the *beginning* of the end, the most important part so look up/savor it friends.

I never remembered your sins I just put you onto the next lessons. Lord

The decades of people-invasion weren't karma but lessons re: boundaries, wall/locked gate, assertion.

When you discipline children you hurt their feelings in the short term so they can act right in the future.

Style to the end, amen.

Stop cowering like a crushed person but forge ahead instead confident of God's power over walking dead.

Free willers come up with own thing but I'd rather find the groove the omniscient God designed for me.

Stop gauging self by likes. The mark of a true teacher is how many reject him for the truth so disliked.

ARTS OF PALEO FASTING

Revel in minor problem solving at the end. The bumps in the road, savor em cuz it'll never happen again.

It was such a nightmare I went through but I had to go through it so I forgive all of it--I *must* to stay lit.

When I was younger I lacked the level of health I have now from high boundaries and staying hidden/low.

I just do what I do but what I went through to get here you wouldn't want to.

It's not that you're not finished. It's that you got such a huge handle on it--big chunk done re: increments.

You got the boulder up the hill, now it's just a few more mornings of tedious details so it's greater still.

Take a rest after getting that boulder up the hill. That way you're high as a kite when finally there/thrilled.

Mediation tends to soften people's entrenched positions.

I only have confidence in myself, doing what I gotta do to get around em but expecting nothing from em.

I got the boulder up the hill and perfectly finished last minute details. I'm done, thriving, prepared, no fail.

Gotta know who you are to be a star. Avoid ego--it's *Who's* you are, all glory goes to God the Father.

I don't care how much of % they get of my work as long as they make me rich, my penury is the gist.

Finished the last details and now *really* done. How anticlimactic though, nothing is happenin'.

When I track mind into what they have to say--and altho' it's interesting and ok--it's less than my reality.

ARTS OF PALEO FASTING

Got six books done, catalogued and published but now four more with glory to God.

I made all the work available and don't know what's gonna happen and can't be addicted to results, no ma'am.

Constantly un-track the mind, coming into your own moment where past and future unite in new notions.

With all that work behind me I just wanna retire into the fat moment by desk-clearing and seeking clarity.

Retirement is enlightenment from falling out of structure: that tiresome tracking not the mind of the Lord.

I hereby transcend all political psychology (current events) in favor of my own reality and future suspense.

It's not eldering "work", it's eldering consciousness--*sagacity*--where you return to childhood, free.

Everything was so great in my childhood! Our world splintered in the sixties and we all lost our sanity.

Tho' TV is good it's always lower. Same with videos, other views, people in news, whatever--I'm higher.

A big balloon is my symbol of freedom: flying away from the work done, reveling in great achievement won.

The reason we don't talk is I'll never give you a chance to hurt me again chump.

I know how fast all can fail so I got humility and solid dependence on God: for success set sail.

From a cold heart/seared conscience you're young again, pliable in God's hands, nice but sly as fox.

Let music be your default setting. Always return to calmness, expansive thoughts, confident/happy.

ARTS OF PALEO FASTING

Desire for approval for what you're achieved is a natural and worthwhile goal for in God it was conceived.

Don't worry they get it from what you've already presented--it's done, you've won, retirement is fun.

I'm happy with the quality of my life now and more money won't change that-- it's good to know it.

As one becomes a success the others reject those who haven't made it yet and the result: mental illness.

When the successful one is also evil, the whole clan becomes dispossessed if they worship moneyed people.

When the weasel becomes the king and the superior man remains on the periphery: hell to pay.

I've studied genius and saints all my life. I'm not saying I'm one but there is a hierarchy liberals deny.

I'm always more interested in working than marketing so I ran outa money and there was little/no selling.

Now I've grown up and am reviving all this. I'm leaving a legacy I confess.

Strict routine office hours: Office One, am-noon (with dogs). Office Two: noon-5 pm (with cats to love).

It's the end of a long haul, a monumental achievement so now go slow, be deliberate, take it easy.

Don't fret you didn't follow your plan cuz it's all about God's plan, man! And that's what you've been doin'

Just because they find you unworthy of their attention you desperately want their attention more, amen?

Their cool rejection was the ontologically fatal insight preceding psychotic shock from a family who sucked.

ARTS OF PALEO FASTING

Don't resent past tyrants just see the system that brought it on: you were sick, addicted, negligent, down.

In other words, don't sink in your swill.

You have every right to be proud of yourself for all you've accomplished. SEE this by taking distance!

Six books and 8 long picturestrips to be viewed and enjoyed while you vaca and live off results of your toil.

I did the best I know how, and I was driven. Though fired by neurosis/need for attention I did it/I'm retirin'

Not just need for justified recognition but driven to know my Self and all God had been pre-designin'

I can see it happening---a giant deja-vu. I knew it in my mind's eye--always working towards it, whew!

Anyone can look you up, that's the point. So just make your books available then wait/have a joint.

I want it all behind me though, the intense focus/work load. I want to open up, take distance, relax ya know?

In all fields it's the same thing and process. Seed, germination, completion: had a guess/overcame mess.

Tho' all they did was try your patience, reward people for trying. With poor character though, fire em.

Let it occur while you detour: the explosion from your work. You were sent by God, it fits this era perf.

You worked but also waited--you were patient, man! Not many worthless accomplishments but One.

What a thrill it is to be done, as completion is part of nature! I'm exalted as my eyes go to the future.

ARTS OF PALEO FASTING

You planted a helluva seed, I'm mean it's *huge*. Now just wait for the inevitable to occur and get ready too.

It's all gonna happen just like you always thought. You had a lifelong vision and it was God you sought.

I love to think futuristically--outa the present box, to be free: fantastic productivity and money.

No matter how good it is it's lower than my own reality so why bother, just proceed so they're freed.

Your own personal reality is hard-won because it means overcoming the scum of social hypnotism.

Exhausted scientist said "Now I'm old, now it's happening but that's the way things go undoubtedly."

B. LASCIVIOUS LIBERALISM

Those who hate the truth call truth "hate".

I judged myself through their eyes. They saw me as insignificant, replaceable, not worth a cent.

It's not science it's a fad, and mental illness is not a civil right.

Not just Obama but an entire generation who supported him. He was smooth and they were lulled.

The nitpicking and scrutinizing for offense is now getting much more intense.

Culture is falling into chaos and debauchery like old civilizations in bible filled with monsters and murder.

Be careful of "gay Christians" or "gay conservatives" cuz they are activists when it comes to their "issue".

ARTS OF PALEO FASTING

The second amendment is our immune system against tyranny so that is why we defend it like crazy.

Unhinged, deranged leftists driven to insanity by a lying left-wing media feeding the frenzy on a daily basis.

Not "news" but smearing innocent people while encouraging mass hysteria and violence in left-wing lunatics.

Media driving America into a bloody civil war in their desperate attempt to destabilize the nation.

Let's get em shooting in the streets then call in UN "peacekeeping" troops, depose Trump, disarm pop.

No more public speaking if you can't monitor the crowd. In the good ol' days people were decent/mild.

Conservatives must start thinking about security. Never go to restaurants or places without it, surely!

The kids are told "everything fun in life is illegal, immoral or fattening". So do whatever you want Kathy.

Discover what your child is being taught (and groomed for) to accept as "normal, good and natural."

Dems desperate Kavanaugh will tip the balance so they can't kill babies anymore and thus their tactics.

The cold dems wanna maintain sexual irresponsibility by killing babies when it comes to Roe vs. Wade.

Gang rape allegations: If this is how the dems act outa power how would they act in/with Hillary Clinton?

The huge gay lobby is constantly ranking the corporations/upping their criteria to avoid prosecution.

ARTS OF PALEO FASTING

Gay lobby long tendrils: They'll monitor a company's gay standards but also those of their vendors.

They're always building the frame of the argument and we're always reacting to the frame and feel framed.

They cut all videos of ex-gays because they "demean homosexuality". The only way out is Jesus, truthfully.

Someone once said "If sodomy's not wrong, nothing's wrong."

America cannot be exceptional if it promotes and celebrates the advancement of the homosexual sin.

Moderates like Dana Perino are socially liberal republicans/increasingly going along with the gay plan.

These liberal moderates are openly trying to make the republican party pro-homosexual like it's swell.

Growing LBGT tyranny is swallowing us/every institution up like quicksand or a cobweb/we're sick of em.

In the name of non-discrimination, they discriminate. In the name of civil rights, they take away rights.

Sin is never on the "right side of history" because it transgresses the design of the Creator of it all, God.

They can't fill desires with God so there's a restlessness there and perversions are always expanding.

They're nurturing homosexual identity and since behavior flows from identity they do bathhouses/disgusting.

Left: performance anger, destruction theatre or inciting violence against those who hate their behavior.

This isn't a war with a front you can see, but a bunch of weasels and losers sniping behind the scene.

ARTS OF PALEO FASTING

End Transgender Tyranny.

Estrogen turns the man into a handicapped man and the testosterone in the woman to a handicapped man.

Oppose transgender child abuse.

People for traditional values have become second class citizens under the law as they hammer in anti-God.

The Sexual Revolution is a totalitarian ideology--it relies on *force*. It's not for Christians of course.

The church needs to help homosexuals but not concede and cave in to gay activists/let their stuff in.

Grotesque/well-coordinated character assassination by democrats and "Dr. Ford" raised a mil to pay for it.

Geo Soros sends 246 million to pro-abortion groups to smear Kavanaugh. Thought he was behind it.

When liberals replace you easily the message is you're not worthy and if you're not sure of yourself, bye bye.

Their cool rejection was the ontologically fatal insight preceding psychotic shock from a family who sucked.

Confusion: We were always told racism is of the far right but now liberals are loudest against whites.

We're entering most prosperous times in America and it makes the Trump haters even more enraged at ya.

Liberals used to say don't judge by skin color but now it's all they do as they try to aggravate a race war.

Love can only beat terrorism if it has lots of guns. Would it have worked with Hitler? Of course not hon'.

ARTS OF PALEO FASTING

Main shovedown since kindergarden: "We're all one" and it's B.S. hon'!

Lack of rationality is too much for me. Calling anyone who thinks differently a racist and they believe it.

Feeling of being censured and misjudged is so breathtakingly appalling it's not worth it staying in the ring.

They are so creepy as through social hypnotism they believe what they're saying and it's frightenin'

The more progressive ideologue Millennials take over the more I just wanna get away/ the heck outa here...

There's a callousness to you guys. You think you're not callous but you're the most callous of ever.

It's just too eerie being banned, censored and scorned. This isn't America it's a progressive hell adorned.

Don't shudder as thou looks back. It was wisdom from age you lacked when you had the herd's back.

You literally didn't know what you were doing. That's what Lord said as demons blinded/made us lowly.

When liberals replace you easily the message is you're not worthy and if you're not sure of yourself, bye bye.

Simply put: The reason we love him is the reason they hate him. That's how wide the gulf is again.

Because they follow the narrative not bible they just mumble and stutter trying to explain their behavior.

Yes you were a sinner and that's why they turned on you but it gave you a view of their utter badness too.

The bible is the central document of western culture, defining truth and how we should act (mature).

ARTS OF PALEO FASTING

Inequality of Outcome is always blamed on patriarchy or whitiies. Never IQ, the reason for discrepancy.

Obama was pro-war yet--unbelievably--all anti-war protests from the left stopped/wanted power more.

Obama spent 1.6 million restoring graffiti of communist dictators. Che Guevara, Castro and other traitors.

Obama tried to outlaw family farms, raising the demand for illegal immigrants (we were alarmed).

Since most criminals are black, Obama said it's racial discrimination to not hire criminals, imagine that.

Under Obama Americans on food stamps went from 33 to 49 million, beginning the homeless problem.

They don't want massive immigration cuz they love em but to change society by destructive savagery.

People don't hate immigrants they don't want their society to change--our traditions/bible, deranged.

Hillary, Barrack and Megan all grandstanded using a tragedy to put their own agenda out--disgusted.

Democrats will always use a crisis to grandstand, ever taking advantage of the opportunity but a funeral? Really...

Just like Italians suddenly reversed against Mussolini, it's happening suddenly against Obama, the creep.

And we're sick of all the gratuitous sex on TV too.

Hollywood awards viewers down 20% last year. We're sick of the hatred and Trump smears.

They're mad Donald was golfing during funeral but he was not invited, so what do they expect, ya know?

ARTS OF PALEO FASTING

Bowed his head to Jesus, He stood for Uncle Sam, he only loved one woman and proud of all he had.

Our sweet life suddenly changed thru regulation. We feared a knock at the door, a police state nation.

The eight years of hell Hussein Obama brought on us: The police state, the fears, the frustrations.

Truth only comes from unbridled speech. Straight from the cuff, fearless, shameless, guilt-free.

Most churches are forsaken, cumbay, false doctrine, filled with demons/no bible.

I came from a blue state. When I realized it was liberalism creating treachery and hate, I escaped.

Believe in somethin'--even if it's a lie, believe in it! Colin Kaepernick

Everybody and their mama having babies outa wedlock and the preacher don't say nothin' about it.

Equality is a dangerous myth.

Civilized restraint is the antidote to chaos.

Who is supercilious? The leftists. We as conservatives just wanna be left alone and we're serious.

They pour out arrogant words, speaking hard things: all the evildoers boast loftily. Jude 14, 15

LGBT Agenda snuck into "Character Education".

School book "Marked" describes having sex in the hallways or with students, now common incidents.

Fallen false preacher going along with LGBT agenda: "I would rather err on the side of love, not truth."

ARTS OF PALEO FASTING

They want you to look the other way so that they can do as they see fit with you and your children.

I'm not against pronouns I'm against legislation about what words I can utter.

The gender pronouns required are artificial constructions of radical ideologues whom I do not respect.

Kindness is always the excuse when the SJW's wanna control what people think, say, do and support.

The highest value is TRUTH not "kindness".

Kindness means supporting perverts.

SJW's aren't motivated by "kindness" but *power*.

As a result of Obama's hustling white people are hated more today than anytime in the world's history.

Police officers are under attack more today than anytime in American history due Obama's treachery.

Undermining our alliances, cozying up to Russia--what happened to our republican party? Obama

Reps aren't cozying up to the KGB, it's just more lies. If you want you doctor you can keep him, relax.

If they make a mistake I don't want them punished with a baby. Barrack Obama

80-90% of black people voted for the son of Satan twice. And you say they're victims and nice?

Obama overturned "Don't ask, don't tell" in the military and since then gays run around visibly and clearly.

You must conform exactly to what they're saying or you're on the other side and they're complaining.

ARTS OF PALEO FASTING

Longwinded narcissist thinks his every word is gold when just by his loquacity it's all bull.

Identity politics is the politics of our time, the refuge of the scoundrel and blind boastful twitter hater.

When calling someone "racist" the power lies with the accusation not the facts.

Conservatives vs. liberals. As we toughen up they just get weaker. They can't answer questions/cheaters.

Victim politics is the curse of our time, the excuse of scoundrels.

Invaded by kids born in the sixties and man oh man did they make me crazy as I learned about boundaries.

To have equal outcomes you'd have to have heaviest bureaucracy possible and that means ending it all.

Querulous self-righteousness combined with refusal to look inward to motives is characteristic of this age.

New lesson from Serena incident: You cannot criticize a prominent black person without it being "racist".

Same enemies/same friends: shifting coalitions is what makes the soaps run.

Black on white violence is unreported, you don't say it. Things are building so a knock on your door, fear it.

Bible reports societies filled with monsters and freaks so evil endlessly and God said kill em all please.

These days if you're smart they'll beat you up (don't understand you) so don't expect approval til' through.

An all black school is called a prison.

When I think all that I went thru being looked down on, disassociated and rejected by liberals.

ARTS OF PALEO FASTING

I didn't leave the left, the left left me. Black Pigeon

The politics of redistribution was replaced by the politics of recognition: my *identity*, who I am.

America's identity went from inclusion to division: demanding respect for oneself as different.

Modern Socialism get-it: it's not for middle class but identity politics around which all else orbits.

They battle in the Oppression Olympics over which group is least privileged and aren't we sick of this?

To today's left, blindness to group identity is the ultimate sin.

In the left's destructive crater identity politics and oppression olympics spiraling is at the very center.

The left's exclusionary identity politics is ironic since their whole thing was inclusion, a big problem.

We love and trust Trump not listening to fake news chumps.

Democratic Socialism is nothing but Socialism with a nice word in front of it. Ben Shapiro

If everyone's doing "social justice" stuff how do you stand out doing crap like that? Be unique/get clout.

Abused for years by liberals in small desert town: a nightmare against conservatives you see all around.

Buy Karen Kellock Books: Amazon. There's 10+ there: early works from 2004 and now five more, mature.

C. FRIGHTENING FEMINISTS

Main gist of feminism: Men and women are the same but women are better.

ARTS OF PALEO FASTING

Wiping out all differences between men and women is a social imperative cuz One-Ism triggers feminists.

Gist: Any differences between men/women (or races) are socially constructed and therefore *unjust*.

Women think they're not sinners. It's all the men ya' know but they're ruined by this lack of humility, utters.

Marriages break up at 6/10ths but when I broach the subject I'm banned from list if it's filled with feminists.

"I can't specifically say that he was one of the ones who assaulted me"--after accusing him of gang rape!

Key accuser backtracks on charges: "I don't know what he did". Another bites the dust: women are liars.

The false accusers--FEMINISTS--will soon fall flat on their face cuz the world is sick of these antics/disgrace.

I'm interested in men cuz they're different from me. How they know all about engines/tools fascinates me.

Men are so logical and sweet--they just wanna please! But then there's the feminist/bitchy wannabes.

God purposefully put me in hard gnarly situations so I could solve them and then write all about em.

I could write about failed feminism to fill a library cuz I had two older feminist sisters tyrannizing over me.

My mother gave up her morals and religion to maintain relationship with my sisters: liberals and fems.

To be in conflict between right and fitting the blight she had to drink, daily-- that was the secondary tragedy.

From resisting losing her culture she "loved the whole world" then got drunk daily to submerge the slur.

Liberal feminists hate the conservative lady in their family. She puts everything they think crazily in jeopardy.

Women were supposed to take care of the children or write hymns not preach fem/Jezebel doctrines.

Jezebel is man-hating (makes em into wimps with bickering) and that's why it hates Trump, rebelling.

When women exit the haze of Jezebel Feminism they think the opposite to everything they did.

Most of the problems we have to day are created by optimists.

6500 genetic differences between men and women--how could anyone say they are the same or even similar?

Stay away from me you grabby, gabby Jezebel.

Men and women are the same: all differences are socially constructed and need to be wiped out/tamed.

He-she wrestler beat female opponent so bad her career ended--and we're supposed to be ok with this.

They say there's no binary since there are intersex people. Deconstruct: This is all political to screw us up.

Non-binary is anti-male just as diversity is anti-white.

There were a few good members but basically run by females and they were uncaring, vapid, tough, cruel.

Be under a woman tyrant and you'll wish it was a man cuz they've had centuries to temper power man.

ARTS OF PALEO FASTING

Women are choosing to raise children without fathers. Of course, men in general are shoved asunder.

Violent, alcoholic and schooled in psychological terror she sure doesn't seem to be a natural mother.

Good housekeepers are "obsessive compulsive"--beginning with Harriet Craig (1949) movie brainwashing this.

Jezebel: Given a chance she'll take your stuff, your boyfriend, your friends and your good reputation.

Men are so much better at being female athletes. And beating them--in fact they knock em out/cheat.

She smashed her racquet on the court but she had many cuz they're used to this kinda crap of course.

See what liberal feminism does? She'll go down in history as a crazy feminist/tennis genius.

"You owe me an apology—say you're sorry" wow we're really seeing 30s-something immaturity.

For years she thought she was supposed to be angry all the time--her favorite phrase was "I'm furious".

"If I could I would take this f-ing ball and shove it down your f-ing throat". Serena Williams to linesman.

"Men do things much worse than that--this is *not fair*". Wow, I've heard that before from the immature.

"Other people were speeding too, officer" yah but you were the one pulled over.

After throwing an ugly tirade "I'm here fighting for women's rights, equality and all kinds of stuff". Yuk

Fight for women's rights by refusing to be subject to the rules they agreed to, yah that's them alright.

ARTS OF PALEO FASTING

Women's Rights: The right to not be subject to the rules you agreed to.

A "feminist" who has been incredibly cruel to other women in the sport.

You must push back against verbal abuse of judges because if it ever worked it would escalate with jerks.

Serena to the linesman: "Are you the one who screwed me over last time? You're ugly on the inside".

Saying "those shouldn't be the rules" doesn't change the rules. That's why you're paid millions, fools.

Which proves being filthy rich with millions of fans doesn't make you a mature or even a nice woman.

It will come out--your immaturities will be shouted from the rooftops!

PRO TENNIS CHANGES AS FEMINISM DERANGES IT

Female empowerment apparently means not having to play by the rules you agreed to.

Men have to play five sets, women only three. But they got equal pay anyway, for 60% of the work, see?

Women size each other up and bash em down. Don't discuss your plans with em it's only God's plan.

Men have learned thru the centuries how to temper power, keep their enemies closer or transmute fear.

How can you watch NFL when you have Women's Tennis, the real sport of men?

Now is the time for the fake feminist showdown. Women have it all wrong and men must now show them.

The linesman didn't "steal a point from her" but made her accountable for her actions.

ARTS OF PALEO FASTING

To not criticize Serena Williams because she has ovaries and dark skin is the very definition of sexism.

Lord, how long will the wicked triumph and exult? Psalms 94: 3

Men are so much better at tennis it isn't funny yet the media says that's a sexist comment/can't face reality.

Two feminist sisters who totally rejected me/conservatism as stated here and thus my drive to be up there.

A loving home is a touch of heaven until degraded into hellhole sewer by feminist leaven.

Women are supposed to be keepers of the hearth, to hold things high and keep the bad out, bye bye.

They're so sweet when they go off to college but then arrogance takes over and a Jezebel Spirit/deranged.

It wasn't a temperment breakdown/disgustingly infantile reaction it was "fighting for women's rights".

Yes she abused her racquet but Ramos abused his authority. Women's Tennis Association Racket

Modernization of sports replaced the classical notion of "virtue" with the modern one of political correctness.

They now use sport to promote feminism, multiculturalism, ethno-nationalism or sexual identity.

The stellar virtue of classical athleticism is now replaced by the pseudo virtue of victimization.

Pathetically infantile behavior is now transformed into the greatest valor.

An embarrassing adult temper tantrum is all-ok if it stands up for political correctness.

ARTS OF PALEO FASTING

Instead of promoting virtue/self-control their sport's used for feminism, multiculturalism, sex identity.

So-called virtue of feminist-inspired equal rights justifies acting out in the most absurd tantrums/fights.

Having been placed in absurd liberal feminist drunken environment I built muscle/could write about it.

Serena Williams meltdown is a public demonstration of just how morally vapid political correctness is.

Naomi is the true champion, showing respect for her opponent while her opponent only herself.

The 3 R's: Rights, Respect and Responsibility means filthy pornographic Sex Ed starting in kindergarden.

"Gender expression" is one thing: fashion. It's how you present yourself in public not victimization.

So now fashion-criticism will be a hate crime.

With millions riding on the game you think judge-abuse is rare? They gotta be strong/ignore the dare.

Women should be able to break all the rules they themselves agreed to. This is all bull/ typical of females.

When the richest most powerful athlete has a tantrum it looks to them instead like obvious racism/sexism.

Incredibly but predictably the lilberal women are bedding down migrants. No kidding, this is serious.

Women hold each other down like crabs in a bucket and I'm telling you I'm sick of it. Ignore em/fu**it.

Fat women, dumb women, dumpy/old women are bedding down migrants who are happy to oblige em.

ARTS OF PALEO FASTING

Once the evil Jezebel spirit is gone thru knowledge alone everything comes into divine order once again.

Loving home is a touch of heaven but when it's leaven and feminists dominatin' it's a hellhole of shoutin'.

Dumpy middle aged women having sex with handsome migrants who can see thru em and are using em.

It was so horrible to be under a liberal feminist I can't even describe it: the illogical flipflops/I defied it.

Pocahontus Fullashit continued liberal tradition of <u>just making it up</u> for Harvard University professorship.

A good housekeeper is thorough: *behind and under!*

Migrants have become boy toys for leftist menopausal women? Yes sir and they'll even travel for it.

Women act like crabs in a bucket when they get with each other so just walk away even if it's mother.

You don't respond with joy just because you can't handle negativity in your life.

Anger and resentment can be Defending Moral Values and love and forgiveness don't belong here Sue.

Since they can't handle negativity everything is good. It's all virtue signaling but through hearts of wood.

It's not men holding women down! Like crabs in a barrel they do that themselves and it's cruel.

Women think "love and kindness"--not truth--comes first. Would kindness with Hitler have worked?

Middle aged liberal women are bedding down migrants and that's a fact overlooked about sluts.

ARTS OF PALEO FASTING

Virtue signaling, kindness without repentance and other women tendencies have cruel outcomes believe me.

Many of the "champions" self-indulge in virtue signaling to distract from their poor performances.

Crazy women forcing veganism on their poor dogs, cats and children--all because they "love them".

Radical feminists have lost the plot. They are very pugnacious, heck in the 80's they were beating me up. Start

I revel in being a woman as that's what God has assigned me--tho' logical it's the humble feminine.

The price of endlessly appealing to female vanity is anti-male sentiment. Stefan Molyneux

I hereby will not talk, discuss or argue with liberal feminists ever again cuz as long as they're one it's sin.

A crappy mother relationship ruins your life but God gives another chance: forgive her/no more strife.

Here I was, an anchor in the mud for my sister's virtue signaling and it lasted for years: my neurotic tragedy.

The daughter was unconsciously being used to dampen the Nazi guilt of the parent, also abused.

Two lesbians who had a son who turned out to be trans, oh what a surprise.

A simple reprimand becomes bullying or misogyny with feminist babies.

Serena took the two components of identity politics: black and female. An atom bomb but she still lost/failed.

Pulled the female card and cried on the court, starting a social justice tirade while the crowd roared.

ARTS OF PALEO FASTING

It's incredibly sexist and racist to excuse her bad behavior because she was black or female.

Black women lack the emotional fortitude to keep their cool in tough situations so we should pity them?

Pitying them rather than expecting better is the *bigotry of low expectations*--like with Serena it ruins em.

Racquet-smashing and crying victim is fighting for women's rights.

Most of the problems we have to day are created by optimists.

Non-binary is anti-male just as diversity is anti-white. Men turning feminine, women just bright.

I judged myself through their eyes. They saw me as insignificant, replaceable, not worth a cent.

There were a few good members but basically run by females and they were uncaring, vapid, tough, cruel.

Be under a woman tyrant and you'll wish it was a man cuz they've had centuries to temper power man.

Anything can replace anything and it will be the same. That's interchangeability, the concept of the lame.

D. HOSTILE INVASION OF YOUNG MEN

Why *must* we embrace large numbers of people so unlike ourselves? No other race is ever asked this.

They want em coming very fast in large numbers cuz that WILL bring change, not tiny groups assimilating.

Marxism and communism was done in the name of equality then hundreds of millions people were dead.

ARTS OF PALEO FASTING

Low openness associated with high orderliness is interpreted as "disgust" and I can say that it sure is.

Low Openness combined with High Order equals Disgust.

They tie our hands behind our back while handing the EU a baseball bat. European citizen

It's all due to Western Ethno-Masochism: white people hating themselves. Why else care more for others?

"Replacism" is the idea of general interchangeability: that one group equals (same as) another, unbelievably.

NWO: Motive #1 for mass immigration is dissolve nations. Motive #2: use em as social engineers for *change*.

The acceptance of multiculturalism means they also accept international agreements killing nationalism.

Soldiers always fought for independence and democracy by defending their borders, you don't know this?

Equality of Outcome is dangerous beyond belief. It's Robin Hood communism steal your life like a thief.

The demented left helps the rich with massive immigration, internationalism and multiculturalism.

Obama called written tests "racial discrimination" making it simple for foreigners to scam our great nation.

Anything can replace anything and it will be the same. That's interchangeability, the concept of the lame.

We've gotten so bad that open border politicians are actually called "centrist".

Whites have a culture, more than most. Who ever started the rumor we were boring milquetoast?

ARTS OF PALEO FASTING

Create civil war to leave EU dictators in power/army controlling borders: Merkel's Kalergi plan of course.

McCain wanted to turn our great majority white country into just another part of the third world/shoddy.

Whoever wants open borders wants America poor. That is the socialist's plan so they promise more.

A majority white safe place for now, but how long before we too are flooded with strangers we don't know?

200 million people into Europe in the next two decades, mostly from Africa.

Globalism is simply the extent of WWII eugenicist Nazi gone underground.

All who know the joys of freedom are winners. WWII survivor

Young male migrant pushes ahead of an old feeble woman in the food line and the state calls her a "Nazi"

First three issues of future politics: border security, economic security, cultural security—that's it.

There's nothing they can do short of war to stop the nationalist age flourishing all around us: Yes!

Transnational dynamics encouraged mass (massive) immigration having no loyalty to local customs.

Global division of labor: Labor goes to third world and rural screwed as capital finance stays in urban areas.

Rural: Mass unemployment in globalist economies when work goes to poor countries/money goes to cities.

Cruel Events: Globalism's narcissistic/consumer based values replacing timeless customs/traditions.

ARTS OF PALEO FASTING

Matteo Salvini: 70% approval as he gives flat tax to encourage growth and incentivizes high birth rate.

80% of central American women are raped when crossing the border. The families know it/warn her.

China (Chicoms) meddle 1000x more than Russia ever could but the liberals love them/help em.

Anyone not for importing millions of unvetted military age men is an extremist, can't you see this?

Multiculturalism means one thing for sure: the erosion of the culture of the native people made poor.

An ivy league study shows illegal pop is 22 million--twice what they said as if we were brain dead.

In communism you don't work 8 hours a day you gotta be *at* work 8 hours a day producing nothing, ok?

Left has left the middle class behind who want Trump--to remedy they import new voting block.

Merkel madness has destroyed European culture. A merchant of misery a little lower than Uncle Hitler.

They're the shit of the earth--they barbecue live dogs, a curse--and you wanna let em all in/put em first?

It's all due to Western Ethno-Masochism: white people hating themselves. Why else care more for others?

"Replacism" is the idea of general interchangeability: that one group equals (same as) another, unbelievably.

Is it racist against blacks to say they create 500% more crimes than natives? Or immigrants, 4000% more?

Appreciation of freedom is the highest winning. Concentration camp survivor

APPENDICES

Key-Locks

for Daily Fastarians.

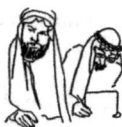

I. How I eat today determines how I'll feel tomorrow.

2. Daily FF Fastarians should feel great as they awake.

3. If I overdo I'll suffer in life, love and looks tomorrow.

4. Self-gentleness from repentance is key: out with shame, in with God's love.

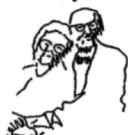

5. I'm cerebetonic with special needs for privacy and solitude.

6. Realizing my uniqueness keeps me in the fast not the past.

7. There is never reason to eat more than once daily.

8. There is direct connection between food and mood.

9. I must fast (on people, habit or food) for success. It's the last piece of my destiny-puzzle.

I0. Fasting overcomes enemies. In rising above fog and frenzy I come inside to Self and God: perfection and protection.

ARTS OF PALEO FASTING

11. Maturity is actions not words. I must do what I say, not say "I will fast" only to eat, cheat or meet with sleaze.

12. Commitment to the fast shows strength, worth and character. I won't give in to fickle feelings for food or fear.

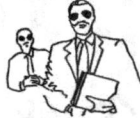

13. Beauty is my duty. By being my best for the rest I'm pure strength and beauty to look up to.

14. Finding myself is very important for mankind. To stay a slob is to rob the mob.

15. It is valuable to learn of my tendencies, talents and terrors. I cannot adapt to people just God.

16. I take my orders from above though it conflicts with man. I seek no honors from men just good reputation with God.

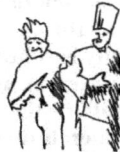

17. Since God is the only source, faith in fickle man is the basis of depression, sin the basis of loneliness and listening to society the basis of bore-dumb. Faith and focus on God is joy.

18. Knowing all men are sinners, I'm untroubled by tribulation. Knowing God as my only Source, man can't take me off course.

19. Problems resolve through prayer and fasting, not looking to man. Advice-taking is life-faking.

20. Fasting days are happiest days. I look forward with glee as it benefits me and brings me closer to Thee.

169

Big Ten

Link to the New Consciousness:
"Lift Off" with Fruit or Fauna

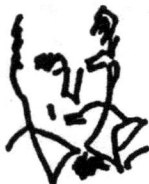

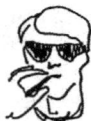

My daily "lift off" is fruit smoothe and before noon lunch. If I fast for the day I know I've eaten the best at the outset. But there are some reclusive types (living in the natural wilderness) who prefer the "trail mix" route—four ounce black fruit, four ounce nuts, two ounce cheese (fauna). It's very French: cheese, nuts and fruit. The higher paleo faster can fast all day on very little of these gut-dense fruity/fatty foods. The grapecure (in the form of raisins) or figs combined with fat can be their daily fasting diet for life. It was mine for five years and I got healthier by the day. My cleansed stomach shrunk to a walnut and I was rarely hungry and when I was just one or two figs sufficed. This is the Queen's Portion—tiny mouse meals. It's a paradox: royalty eats little and walks tall while the masses eat it all missing God's call. It may seem strange but I never craved a thing for just a little fat removed the temptation-sting. If thirsty grape-aid (just a drop of grape in 8 oz water) provided minerals that quench craving for other things. The proportions of figs/raisins to nuts or cheese may change and later reverse back into red salads and fauna.

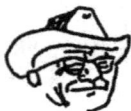

Of course, the fruit-nut-cheese diet arouses so much controversy. "It will cause candida or mucus--the mixture of sweet fruit and cheese". No way, even fruit juice after cheese blends right in and facilitates digestion. It is splendid--the figs eliminate mucus at a rate of 30 (four times eliminative as juicy fruit) and they are filled with iron, potassium and magnesium--bringing blissful feelings and elation. The face doesn't broaden, it narrows--for the tiny bit of cheese streamlines the body and suppresses appetite all day long. The nuts add fiber and colon-happy "higher-paleo" fat for perfect elimination. The combo fills up without filling out like juicy fruit does--it subtracts without adding. Simplicity is the key-note for higher paleofasters along with routine and

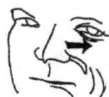

short shopping lists. "We're so sick of so much folderol surrounding food, and things like canned fruit lessens the complexity. We just want our little box of raisins nuts and sometimes cheese purchased anywhere on earth fitting in our pocket or purse. When hungry for more we'll just grill a delicious streak of course."

LESS IS MORE!
Letter from Recovered Ana in France:

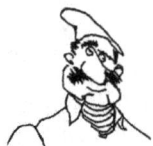

"I could have avoided years of hell had I known about you. I'm out of the hospital and finally my family is able to accept my different diet, since I stay healthy even though thin. Interestingly, eating this way is very French so it was easy—a little cheese and a grape has always been our snack. It makes me so happy living like this, dealing with my full-phobia and being able to trust these foods. They are like power-houses and the usual physical problems of anorexia are eliminated while staying (relatively but not shockingly) thin. I just wish I had known about these neat techniques before I was hospitalized and ruined my family. My French parents understands a diet like this—of raisins, cheese, fruit, nuts, peanut-butter, occasional fish or chicken, a cheese omelet on occasion. And yet still I remain thin enough for my own strict standards—even Hollywood's. Had I known all this I could have avoided anorexic institution hell."-*I.D.N, Paris France*

SpeaKK

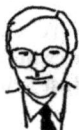

Question: *How do you see present society, as revealed by the reality show fad?* KK: Godless superficiality, gross carnality, crass conformity, obstructive materialism and embarrassing hedonism. It's a sick society and getting sicker every day God is left out. It all started in the public schools and now we've got a nation of not champs but fools. They can't think, having lost that ability in adapting to the New Age reality--taking it all on by rote. Even while they're saying it they know they're wrong but still want to join the throng. These shows are so silly— the participants act like young children in their clowning and chaotic chattering. I long for the old days of perfect productions and stylish exemplars. People now are so steeped in selfish sensuality they brag about the very thing they should be ashamed of. Coupled with this is extreme media idolatry of immoral people. Partying, and anything goes--and look how low they go. Listen to one who knows: God says it's better to mourn and fast than go to the feast in hilarious gaiety. And their laughter sounds like cackling thorns over a fire--you can't trust Joe Party who's really a liar. The latter days are filled with haters of good--they hate "morality" for they love their sins by which they're so distracted the creative never wins. That's why they have no breakthrough and remain has-beens. Of course all this is covered over by a super-"nice" image to appear social and "loving" which is regarded as superior to just loving God, who should come first. The "lover of the people" thing is a fake for when you need 'em they're not there in a shake. See that woman who calls herself a kitten? She's really a snake. The champion must separate himself unto God for the sake of his divine destiny and learning to see through people is what it takes.

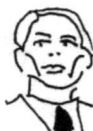

Question: *Can you elaborate on the public schools?* KK: It started to break down in the sixties when moral relativism took over. The NEA controlled by leftist feminist philosophy decided what got taught and it was definitely the witch's philosophy of "do what thou wilt--no moral restrictions". When morality is regarded as intellectually inferior the human tendency is towards concupiscence--fleshy degradation. That's why championship and genius comes from self-restraint which brings humility, while sin strengthens the ego. The former evokes creative action, the latter blocks it. Because they bought the lie people don't know how to think--they just mimic the poli-correct line which deadens their shine. The only solution to social hypnotism is seeking the True Self and God--seek and you'll find. But, we lost our moral compass having swallowed a new reality whole. Practically everyone dropped their guard in the seventies: we couldn't tell right from wrong and many made fools of themselves and the worst cases ended in jail and other ways to fail. An overnight success becomes a shameful failure due to sin and concupiscence--man's tendency towards lust, which ends in self-disgust. Feminists think copying men gives them power but big, loud and mean--not the lady's sheen. The lady is humble and kind, not the social fiend. It's not a true friend, the social scene. And what of promiscuity: this is powerless--not perspicacity. The social soul is filled with the spirits of other people and distractions. He must become pure/not queer to be the seer.

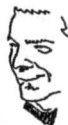

Do you mean we shouldn't trust anyone? KK: Trust no one, bow before no man, seek no honors among men. Jesus couldn't even trust his disciples for he told Peter "before the cock crows you'll have betrayed me three times"--and he did. It's the biggest lesson we came here to learn: Trust only God and yourself, but only after repentance. Previous to that you trust yourself for sin is a possessive force which must be put on the shelf, for the issue is recycled energy in outworn channels which blocks the creative elf.

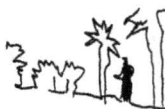

Why do you rhyme? KK: Why not rhyme if that's what you do naturally? If its the truth it should rhyme--for me to not rhyme would be too much trouble. To connect words through not just meaning but sound drives the truth home while opening other levels of thought. Whenever there's a choice between rhyming and not-rhyming, isn't it better to rhyme? It's perfect communication in time. It works on the principal of less-is-more by revealing hidden analogies between the reader and the divine. The rhyme is the tool of the seer--higher poetic images makes one a believer, a discoverer-conceiver. It connects not just *meanings* but *sounds*—this makes higher sense to the human hounds.

.

ARTS OF PALEO FASTING

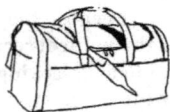

What do you mean "flitting about to little purpose"? KK: This describes post-modernism. Always on the go, ever in contact. Cell phones and cars, only thinking of bars and seldom of Mars. Virtually every disease is caused by self-imposed stress. The immature soul is overextended, to say the least. The most important value of genius is leisure for only in relaxation comes revelation. The neurotic has an incapacity for leisure--though on vacation he is never part of creation--it's just more confabulation (talk) and giving into temptation--a very low vibration. The most productive life is creative work then receiving more inspiration from nature--that's man's highest stature.

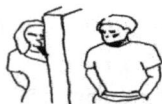

How would you paraphrase the foregoing? KK: Worldliness--mundane, boring, pleasure-and approval-seeking worldliness--is creeping into the churches. Whether churchman or alcoholic, they're all sinners and all must repent lest they stay stressed with the creative all spent.

What is the solution to living amongst all this? Is it wise to know it or would it be better to deny it? KK: It is safe only to be aware of it. To deny it is death--as a victim or in becoming part of it (almost worse than death) for the only way to adapt is to become *dense*. The solution is to fast, find talents and ascend to a higher separate reality from the mass even while still enmeshed.

How do you view your own life? KK: God put me in Paradise so that I could write to those still stuck in swill (like never getting their fill). By staying still, I've become an info-still. Of Godless society and post-modernism I've had my fill.

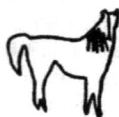

And of modern perversions? KK: The days of Roy Rogers goodness are gone and now perversions and pedophilia fills the vacuum. It is everywhere now and gaining steam. If people are confused they easily fall into deviations of all kinds, limitless. There were nervous fidgeters during the MJ trial--not just predators but the *rank and file*. It all goes with with moral relativism which is the liberal style.

ARTS OF PALEO FASTING

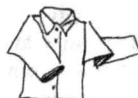

Karen, what are the results of repentance? I'm sure we all know it underneath, but it feels so good to hear someone confirming it. KK: In answer I will give definitions which fit the bill: you get your fill! It is plenary: full, complete. Plenary indulgence: A remission of the entire temporal punishment due to sin. Plenary inspiration: inspiration in all subjects dealt with. Plenipotent: Powerful, most potent, plenipotentiary. Plenipotentiary: lucrative investment with full power. You'll need a person and a diplomatic agent invested with full power to transact your world business. Plentiful: containing or yielding plenty, abundance. Fruitful. Characterized by or existing in plenty. And, although we don't need it the repentant gets a Plethora: fullness, to be full and over-full. A condition characterized by marvelous excess, or superfluity: We have all that we need and more to give away. But to stay replete, the recipient can't be a louse but as humble as a mouse. For it's a sin to reward bad acts like the continuously mildly soused.

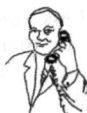

You seem to spend much time in the hot desert sun. Aren't you afraid of skin cancer? KK: No, for skin cancer comes from wrong starchy low-fat diet. The sun-drenched tanned champ gets high-fat and the skin likes/needs that. But the starch-stuffed cell crumples under solar radiation resulting in a mass of wrinkles. The fat-faster may enjoy God's sun, free of fear--let our natural diet dry your tears.

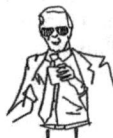

Can you speak on wealth and jealousy? KK: Wealth is not a sign of God's grace since the devil promises it in return for going with him. Wealth can be a consolation cuz he's going to hell for eternity. The bible says don't covet the sinner who is flourishing because soon his day is coming. But God doesn't want us poor and you should repent for more.

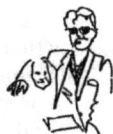

What about your photo-phobia? KK: Taking photos of someone is a severe invasion of privacy--the worst. Pictures are permanent, and no one is perfect 24-7-365. Never let anyone take your picture unless you ask them to--if they do, break the soul-snatching contraption (but pay them for it, too). If anyone underhandedly brings a camera in it's an offense--like other modern inventions it invites pretense. The last time someone came here and surreptitiously took my picture was the last time. But I use it as the only one--for all other picture-taking I'll shun.

ARTS OF PALEO FASTING

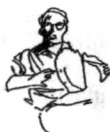

And humility? KK: There would never be an "I" without a God saving me from the whole mess: even while in sin He gave me perfect mercy nonetheless. To my heavenly father I throw a kiss for any wisdom comes from Him (who leaves nothing amiss). Like if I have a whole complex document to correct, He spot-lights the error. If I then laboriously go over the whole thing, thinking "there must be more to this thing, since the error was the first thing seen" it's wasted effort for there never is. The Lord makes my yoke easy, He makes my heart sing. There is no more "I", except the "I" I am in Him. But I stay humble around people because they'll crush you down if you aren't. I am careful to avoid any more of their insults.

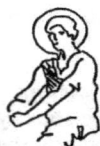

What movie shows most clearly the moral degeneration of new society? KK: *Bully.* If you can stomach it, it shows how social hypnotism and peer pressure ruins lives in the youth generation. Get past the shock to the deeper meaning of this movie and you'll be even more shocked. Then think back to kids you knew like this in high school--usually the most popular. And then realize how much bullying you witnessed--against the shy, the inner, the creative, the ectomorphic, the cerebrotomic. And then realize how such bullying was group-determined (in *Bully*, two of his killers didn't even know him). Many say *Bully* isn't a good barometer--since "they're not all like that". Well, not "all" but maybe many? Bullying is common through soul-murder and exclusion. God was taken out of the schools, and without God one is sucked into worldly wickedness or witchcraft. If most aren't as bad as these kids, most tolerate that social milieu which brings acceptance.

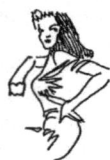

What are the specific signs of false religion? KK: It's wherever New Age fallacies have seeped in and it's all for show. I would narrow it down to two basic heresies: (1) word-and-faith--that we can have whatever we want by our *words* (not necessarily repentance of relationship with God) . Implied here is that man is bigger than God--that he can push Him around as a gift-dispenser. This runs counter to the definition of God as sovereign and omnipotent. The biggest mega-million dollar churches are word-and-faith heretics. It gives people false hopes--that they can have it all without repenting of the sins they love--rather than learning the ropes (fasting, and repenting for joy everlasting). People are gullible because they want so badly to believe they don't have to repent. Along with this is the heresy that God loves them no matter what they do. This isn't true--he hates workers of iniquity, especially those misleading His flock. Psalms says we are to hate what He hates and hate those who hate Him. Psalms 139: 21

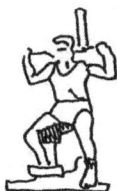

(2) No need of repentance. "Repentance" implies there is sin which is politically incorrect—in the New Tolerance we're supposed to accept everyone and everything—it's all about inclusion. Preachers care more about not offending their tithing congregations than saving them from torment. Their weekly sermon should be to repent, for to sin is to miss the mark (of your highest calling) but to repent is to hit the bull's-eye. But warnings of sin would offend so their soul can't mend. To gain favor it's the wrong (mild, acceptable, palatable) message they send. The prophets and disciples in history were hated, killed, mocked, tortured because they told the truth. That's another way of saying: if you're loved by all you're probably false--you want their approval, even the louse. Is it any wonder the culture is degrading as true glory and godliness is fading? It's our purity of heart which changes God's mind--not our words. This kind of thinking is like voodoo, laced with New Age positivism and self-esteem therapy putting man on top and leaving God out of it. It's all the same mind-game and it means fame for preachers who attract but never—for God says only *repentance* removes symptoms: give up sin, the symptoms leave.

Karen, do you go to Church? KK: No, I avoid gatherings due to MCS but also the churches have changed. From outright heresy to modern sociability seen as godliness and acceptance of compromise. Home is where I gain strength. This is a new society creeping into the churches--more worldliness, confusing sociability with Godliness, virtue signaling with reality. The churches have changed, some becoming deranged. As long as churches are a social thing, it is churchism--the devil's fling--the sanctuary of demons. So cerebrotonics become Christian mystics in desert solitude. All great prophets spent decades in their desert sabbatical alone—then their star finally shone--but in civilization they just groan. Like one Calvinist writer said: "The typical local church either bores me to tears or causes me to lose my composure, exciting rage within my soul. I stopped pew-warming years ago, and just hold Bible studies whenever the Lord leads". This is the exact sentiment of the famous saints in history, according to William James (*Varieties of Religious Experience*).

ARTS OF PALEO FASTING

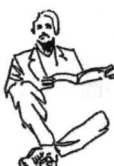

Karen this is fascinating! And so relieving. Would you call yourself a misanthrope--do you hate people? KK: Absolutely not. I'm no misanthrope, but all men are sinners. Knowing that and expecting nothing, I can just be cordial. But putting "love and kindness" before truth (like women do) is dangerous! Women basically know nothing about politics—just the narrative which they chirp. The most important thing seems to be virtue signaling about their goodness but like in the case of open borders, caring nothing about what it does to the people already here—us! They tend to forgive without repentance, creating criminals and recividism. They don't see themselves as sinners and will rail in anger against anyone close. Women need wisdom not viscious feminism. Virtue signaling sends a smug thrill up their spine.

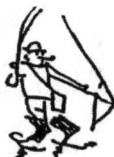

Karen, why do you say one of the most important things about championship is patience? KK: There are patterns: some people had hits and became radically successful after years of tedious and thankless work. Others did two or three titles of their work (albums or books) before they made it. The first two didn't sell but the third hit--then everyone bought the first two. So be patient! Keep doing it: working, fasting and repenting so you may start attracting. Never get dis-couraged--it may be around the next bend, when you've hit the right blend. Just wait and relax but don't get lax.

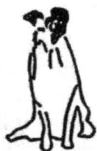

What happened in your case when you repented? KK: I was so happy then and as Sinatra sang, "it's better than coke". Life was a dark, cold, dangerous joke and repentance turned I it all around and everything fit perfectly again as God removed the yoke. The minute I cut all bad associations there was brightness, cheer, purpose because bad links are sin. This is all a wonderful fantasy--you must create the new reality *by* repentance then it will happen: when God wills, it's you He fills. It's all a matter of timing, the blank entry of that for which you've been priming. Starting the new inning is all about the cessation of sinning, then you're ready to grab the gold ring (when in comes around again) and this chance date in history becomes your new fling.

ARTS OF PALEO FASTING

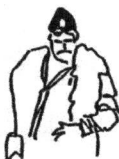

MCS, Multiple Chemical Sensitivities: Can you elaborate on this please? I am also sensitive and people think I'm faking it. KK: I know, people think you're a liar so you can't get well until you put out this fire. People think you're faking being sick around chemicals, civilization or cars--because *sometimes* you can tolerate it. They can't see it's a sliding variable, a matter of TOTAL LOAD from all fronts, effected by diet, environment, situation. Thus immunity is always changing/endlessly mutable so people think you're a hypocrite because sometimes you're sick and sometimes you're not when in the same situation. They'll even "test" this with cruel antics. Like when I was driven up the grade I was so sick the driver had to stop every half mile. But coming back I wasn't sick—infinite variability from the "total load" of immunity. It could have been I was so anxious/glad to be going home, or the air was cleaner at that point, or I was adapting. But evil helpers will sense deception and then: your isolation—sick of defending yourself against accusations of malinguering. Even best friends and family will show understanding but then at times fall back into mundaneity and everything's 0k when it's not mentality. This kind of thing is very trying on spouse and family and only the most empathic can stand it. It's hell living with the general malaise--dizziness, ooziness, everything twirling around--the feeling of extreme car sickness. It is motion sickness like Menier's Disease--even a swing brings on this spinning effect, an hypothalamic thing. Every time a neighbor (even far away) burns trash or lights up their grill with lighter fuel it's a sick night. Only the wealthy can go way out, 100 acres at least. But one can start by putting air filters in *every* room.

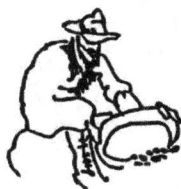

Where did all this begin? In most case candida and low immunity comes from early drugs, antibiotics or even being zapped once chemically. It also can come from early drug or alcohol addiction. Having MCS forces you into a crystalline compactness with everything from routine to staples and that marks the superior man. It isolates you, a very healthy thing. It forces you into your own journey and comfort just to get through the day.

ARTS OF PALEO FASTING

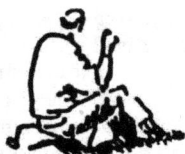

How has feminism affected men? KK: Most men under 50 are beta males having been raised by angry feminist mothers. They transfer this to their wives and follow them like little puppies. Many men are feminine, having lost identification with their fathers and taken on their mothers. And thus starts all the sex role and gender confusion. Add to that dominating angry feminists who have accepted the anti-male narrative and you get one horrible first date or relationship. It's so sad men can't take the lead anymore. And if there's any disagreement whatsoever her femme friends advise her to "get him" and what happens to men in divorce courts is appalling. The education and criminal justice systems are anti-male and in many states she can cry rape two years later, and *many* women use false accusation of child or domestic abuse after which the man's life is ruined forever. Simply put, men have become afraid of women, partially from the mother transference, more from the great danger of false accusation or vindictiveness, but also not wanting to be alone when she's socially skilled or accepted. Male Feminists often turn out to be sadists, since they've accepted the false narrative, given up all their own prerogatives and stood up for the intolerable just to be functional—but every internal conflict based on a lie will eventually burst against the perpetrators/the female snide. What man would want to be around this anti-male thing, being called macho just for having male interests or logical responses? Women have become dominant (no more sweet lil' ladies) and most men don't want that except momma's boys and even they eventually get annoyed.

Art & Science Discovery

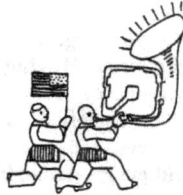

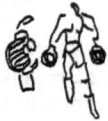

Discoveries are seeing analogies no one has seen before: they have no precedence in the past. The characteristic of all dense environments is contradiction, which is resolved through a Creative Act bridging the gaps and reversing all expectancies. Through unusual analogies, all old molds are scrapped and the real answers are revealed--outside the old frame of reference. In psychology, we look beyond the person and extend our vision to his system to find the answers. In medicine, we look beyond supposed "germs" and genetics to the person's own habits and foods that make him sick. This is switching to a new frame of reference and it always brings the "Ah-Hah" experience of all discoverers and mystics. But to make a real dent, hard science must be presented artistically for the full right-left brain integration (Koestler Structure of Scientific Revolutions, 1962) and thus the Picturestrip as the Superior Instrument was built and demonstrated on www.karenkellock.org.

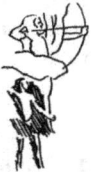

The switch to a new frame of reference is an *invention*, or new world-view. The discoverer does nothing for social approval as everything is written to himself, with only the subconscious selecting and deciding (for only it has tact and delicacy). As soon as the would-be genius listens to others, his virtuosity is lost throwing pearls before swine. When he gets to his highest pitch of self-writing, the most unique becomes the most universal and he becomes an overnight success. When he believes in his work enough (to not have to call someone to tell them about it) it finally comes true.

UNIQUE STYLE: JUST SAY IT

If working only to please the True Self he develops a striking style which is wholly different from the way others think and talk. The lone discoverer is

181

ARTS OF PALEO FASTING

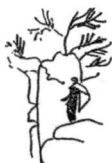

ultra-effective, coming off like a ballad putting science and the world down. This can't come through scholarly authority but through a Creative Act: the right-brain images shoot straight for the heart before "logical argument" can intervene against it, and that's what brings change. Having faced self with no defense and fizzled out with humor, the readers see "all we're doing is useless, or slightly worse than useless." With a laugh of self-derision, the revitalization of culture has now occurred. Since the discoverer puts everything down he puts nothing down and everyone begins to march to a new drumbeat together—this is a Revitalization Movement driving the evolution of history and culture, always led by a charismatic figure like Freud, Jung, Newton, Einstein.

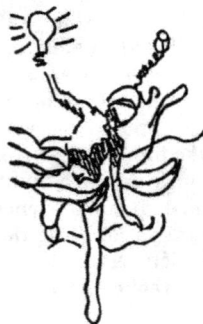

DISCOVERY! If you're trying to be what you are not, you'll never be what you are or what you're supposed to be. The female writer-discoverer who writes about the "land of snobbery and privilege run by the old and silly", or the "stuffy family--a deep conspiracy of silence driven by secret alliances of snooty jealousy" is offending all yet none, for all is "essentially true" yet expressed quickly like a child. The work that loses is the slow, the laboriously detailed showing a lack of self-confidence through loquacity--much too much writing and words. Without self-assurance that *one is right* the language gets tedious, so he says it while avoiding responsibility for saying it by flooding the reader with the nonessential. To be a true revolutionary one must be the most mature which is most simple--then, and only then, can one man be a majority.

FREE SPEECH

We must add to our heritage or lose it. We must go forward not backward by becoming more not less and this all means going towards the self: the pure, unadulterated, persecuted-for-strange-ideas SELF. It's no easy road for the system policy is to wipe out all freedom of the intellect. It matters not what culture it originates in, for all genius discovery collides with acceptable schools of thought and it's chances of changing culture go against overwhelming odds. *Only the True Self--simply expressed--can cut through.*

ARTS OF PALEO FASTING

ONE   BOOK   CHANGES   CULTURE

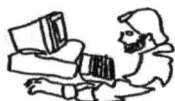

In the hands of the unabashed self, one good book is more effective than war in changing culture. The fate of the world really is determined by poetry, not bombs and bullets! The main gist of genius in all landmark works in history has been hatred of anything authoritarian as he aims all words against cultural prestige. Culture holds creativity hidebound by snobbish tradition, so anyone who has the guts to not need social approval--to break free of this primary tribal need of the human--is "the one" who changes all by producing extraordinary copy that really does change the world.

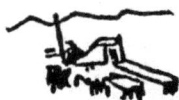

This is not writing to instruct, to bore with descriptions or explanations, but writing for effect. This means austere simplicity, a cute punch with no fear of disapproval or critical rejection. One must have developed his own position without fear of being accused--something taking two to three decades: The inner journey may start at 23 but only at 73 does the sage finally have something great to contribute while being properly armored to prevent a fall. The talents may have been developed quite early in the life but the audacity doesn't appear until far later on, a gift of age when less concerned with peer (vs. sneer) support. One may have shown early talents (the most likely to succeed) yet a decade or two of sin slowed the process while giving them more to write about, to cook in the "slow stew" after the long haul of a starving artist's mining for wisdom.

BEETHOVEN AND BLUE GENIUS

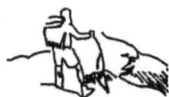

If you will just have the courage to work and wait, fortune will give you opportunity to show your greatness. Looking at great genius in history is instructive: like Beethoven, an ardent, lively temperament of peculiar charm and fervent talent. He was hated by the small townspeople, teased and beaten by children yet was totally accepted by aristocrats at one time, the prince of the city's social life (which he loved)--yet this only happened after his father's death when he was released from family.

183

ARTS OF PALEO FASTING

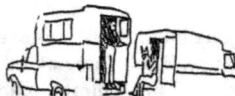

Beethoven was a lone rider on the trail, a genius receiving all inspiration from nature. Despised and ignored at home he became envied by most (a double-edged sword of all gifted people, the biggest obstacle to overcome). He overcame by practicing constantly until he developed a brand new approach to music with dazzling virtuosity and extraordinary skills. Though aging and going deaf he was still filled with youth and the exuberance of his own creative power. When he went deaf he wrote his best and most memorable concerts. He loved society but had to live the rest of his life in solitude. To this he said "Plutarch told me to show defiance to my fate. I shall never crawl. My world is the universe."

INNER POWERS

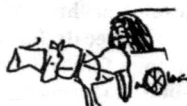

He was a young man with exceptional inner powers choosing to fight destiny, turning fate into his advantage--at which point he became more fervent, more courageous an inventor just as he was no longer able to choose society's glamour. "Where do I get my ideas? Everywhere. Moods translate into words for a poet, or for me, as notes." His true heroism went hand-in-hand with the times: the French Revolution, liberty and equality. He was the first democrat of music--"Heroica" was full of hope for the world. At first he was dedicated to Napoleon until he crowned himself emperor, when Beethoven despised him "as just an ordinary man".

The Age of Enlightenment brings other dimensions to his creativity--a time of stretching human capacity beyond what is comprehensible to others. He said about the Prince: "what you are you are from birth. What I am I made myself. Of princes there are thousands, of Beethoven there is only one!" He loved beauty and romance but despised sensual pleasure for its own sake--loving ancient Greece but hating Rome. The highest romantic sees love as unity of soul and body with God while actual persons he wears as a loose sleeve.

GENIUS IS ALWAYS A PARADOX

ARTS OF PALEO FASTING

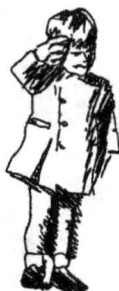

Genius hates any authority other than it's own creative spirit. Beethoven showed a profound yearning for his "other self" which enabled him to endure extreme paradoxes in his life. While at the height of his popularity at age 45 when Kings and Queens celebrated him, he was near poverty. For the next ten years he had more and more solitude--"visitors must write"--and when they came into his presence they had to write conversations in a notebook. His music was so far from his time but so close to us today. The circle of life closes: "an artist never really finishes his work...he merely abandons it." This contradiction--this loner who was worshipped by royalty but hated and violated by townspeople who didn't even know who or what he was-is a great paradox of genius. As Shakespeare said "when beggars die, no comets are seen." But I say repent so your genius comes out and you won't die a beggar. My life's work has evolved to a diamond formula and new matrix for the life sciences:

all success attraction
all disease obstruction
all recovery elimination

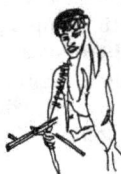

For more on discoveries in all fields, read *Act of Creation* by Arthur Koestler. For no matter what the field there are similar characteristics between all discoverers. They have periods of "fertile anarchy" and "underground games" as the Creative Act matures invisibly. These are the "dry years" of the budding genius--a kind of hell on earth. One must know that the Creative Act is part of nature and it is surely budding underground. You will have your harvest visibly blossoming above ground at the completion of your inner journey marked by highest purity from repentance. Certitude of success is the light guiding you to completion. So just hang on, your time is coming. You might also find Koestler's *Structure of Scientific Revolutions* very instructive, for all discoveries evolve the same way coming through a Creative Act which changes the field every forty years.

High-Fat is High-Tech

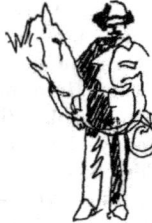

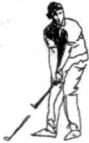

How to hit the bull's eye. Reversal dieting is not about FRUIT or FAT but about the reversals between the two. For some reason that's hard for people to grasp—they want it all-or-none but that's no fun. For when you're under the gun, food won't work. When fruit nor fat works, you must fast and then all the angels are called to oversee your recovery (over your entire situation they lurk). The body is endlessly mutable so you need the fruit-fat reversals and the fast to eliminate the problem (make the system roto-rootable). It's a three-speed diet, and most can eat fruit and fat but not fast (for most, this project comes last). That's ok—just when you're about to give up on D-Day you'll be having a blast. It seems that God puts a thorn in our side until we take the reins and change the tide with the device He created for man: to decrease and go light to be better than before the problem began. You'll love it so much that eating will be like going into a dungeon, through so much pain you've been trudgin.

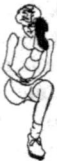

Start to fast and look forward to youthful beauty and happy sagacity until the moment of death. Readers are amazed at their sudden beauty of complexion, newfound energy and clarity of thought (wisdom). Get to know your body and you'll instinctively know when to go fruitarian and when to fat-fast. When I regressed as a fruitarian and suddenly switched to no-carb for one year to revive my protein and fat-deprived system that was the perfect thing to do. I was extremely energetic and happy on a no-carb and fasting diet of just one daily meal of cheese omelet. But then just as suddenly the body said "I want fruit" and now fruit, cheese with nuts worked best followed by light lemon aid for the day. The two sciences below will tailor your choices and temper your taste. But the fast is the point so regarding what to eat don't get out of joint. Just enjoy your life as every

186

ARTS OF PALEO FASTING

moment God anoints, as all food errors the fast offsets (and it never disappoints).

REVERSAL DIETING IS THE POINT

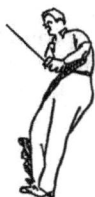

Our perfect diet is endlessly mutable while staying within the general fat-fruit-fastarian matrix. The fruitarian theory says fruit is such a beautifier but yet the elevated insulin brings bloat and bad skin when at a certain stage—when the protein deprivation overrides any benefit from the fruit. It's all a matter of where you're at in the reversal. I choose lacto as home base with fauna later. After so much fruitarian isolation what a relief to feel a part of the world again—to be able to eat most of what my hostess serves yet still have the mysterious highness I crave, fasting later with maximum energy because I'm properly fat-fed.

MAKE THIS DAY DIFFERENT!

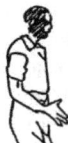

Follow this program and you'll be confident, not shy—for fasting (making a decision and sticking to it) strengthens the will, the self-esteem and self-confidence. Many years ago I woke up to the worst feelings in my life. I was filled with candida, resentment and despair. It was so bad I decided to do the opposite to what I usually do—make it a whole new day, a new stew. I fasted until late afternoon, and the worst day became the best—I started to swoon. I'll never forget that day so remember what I say: Whenever things go wrong, separate from the throng and fast all day long. Stop work, ignore the jerk and get your own Godly perk: fast with God! This is the day you forget the clod and start to look really mod. Just do this once, (it's the last brick in the building) and it'll become your new addiction. Your brand new habit makes you quick as a rabbit. Do it whenever you feel low just to see how high you can go. Can you do it just this day, just once? Never again you'll be seen as dunce. This is the beginning of a whole new life. Nothing hard—just one day fasting is so little to ask so in God's glory you'll bask. I tell you it's just like an old movie—the utter romance of it all and the fabulous detail. And as retained water is rapidly eliminated you'll get as thin as a rail (this divine device will not fail). So when neither fruit nor fat will work, pull your trump card to delete the quirk or gossip by office clerks. For everything they said is now not true—and God knows it, your Avenger so true.

ARTS OF PALEO FASTING

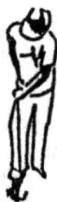

While fasting you come into God's experience. God's ways and thoughts are higher than man's--they are not just *different*, they are *opposite*. Fast, suspend your brain and illuminate. Fast and wait on God--something good's about to happen. Prepare for visitation and your promised rewards, for you're here for a reason—your work is the Lords. The more you fast in optimism the more you'll love doing it and thank God for the privilege of ascension to this greatest spiritual reality. Use this key to victory and experience such great bounty every single day of your long life: the Daily Fastarian is King. Surrounded by gluttons your heart will sing as this divine device conquers everything.

REASONS TO FAST

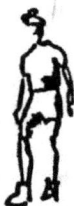

Fasting has miracle power and the benefits are so great you'll be addicted for life. Whenever you hit a glitch, simply switch—to fruit, to fat, or the fast. Fasting, the glory of God will reign in your life. This "day of humiliation" will bring you incredible rewards--"I will increase as you decrease." As you deny your instincts the ego dissolves and the miracle happens: God takes over and gives you all. This sequence has to occur: it is divine law, for to be exalted you must be humbled. To be King you must bow to the floor. To say "I have sinned, so I'll fast and pray" precedes your greatest success. Test me on this. You may have reasons to fast for a special purpose--not to get attention, not to show off, not to brag to the world what you've given up, no announcement--just something between you and God for power and specific solutions. Fast and tell no one. Fast and be silent. The more humble you are the more power you'll have. Though your fast may be mere restriction (just eating less) the rewards are daily and cumulative. A Daily Fastarian is a "mini-faster" and lives in heavenly bliss. We eat one meal (or two) of fruit or fat then we fast 18 hours (God's kiss). No "higher" routine exists for life's a cruel abyss but with daily fasting *nothing's* amiss.

ARTS OF PALEO FASTING

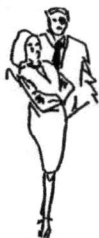

You may be a man or woman of God with real purpose to change society. People are *dying* for what you have. Through fasting (on people, habits or food) the most ugly becomes the most beautiful as all rough edges are smoothed out for success. The way to write, speak or advance a cause is to fast. The silent enemy of your impossible dream is not your mate or lack of knowledge, but lack of fasting. It's time to prune your life in readiness for a blossoming future. Never give up your impossible dream for God will make a new thing: it will spring forth as He makes rivers in the desert. Tighten your belt and it will occur. You must always have faith for the world says you won't make it: *"it's been too long...you're over the hill...you're too old."* Fast and this is false. Shun the cold, go for the gold--just finish your work and do it in bold.

Questions on Fatarianism

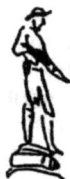

"Won't fat clog my arteries?"

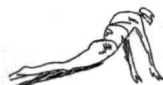

KK: anyone worrying about that has no understanding of the science of metabolism. You know how cats and dogs love fat and practically nothing else? That's the way humans are but the desires are masked with dogma and fear. Only by eating your paleo diet can you prevent being hungry all the time so you can fast for long periods afterward. You take your fat like medicine. I eat raw dairy as a medicine so that the fat will work for me in these ways: appetite suppression, energy, fat-burning, clear thinking and moist skin. This is your regime for your highest scheme: fast at night and in the morning, eat fruit first then your fat and use lemonade for thirst.

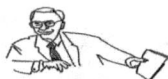

Understand the Science of Metabolism. Cheese only clogs the arteries when mixed with starch. When taken alone, it opens all the arteries, since it elevates glucagons which opens (dilates) everything up and burns fat and cholesterol out of the body. Everyone takes it with starch, so naturally they call it "binding" but if you take things as medicine you never mix them. Cheese without a starch-- enjoy "doughless pizza". Yesterday I ate fish for the protein preceded by fruit. This is Reversal Dieting to constantly be given the benefits of both diets--building up through protein, carving back through fruitarianism and fasting. Fruit or none, that's up to you.

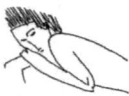

"Sometimes when I eat fruit I feel as big, stuffed and bloated as a cow. And then when I eat fauna, I slim right down again." KK: If you have this reaction you probably have hyperinsulinism (and probably candida) and will really appreciate the dilation

190

and slimming effects of fauna. When you hit a glitch, simply switch and as your IR level changes you'll be able to eat fruit again. I would suggest you switch to non-sweet fruit and have it in the morning (when the reaction is least) and then your fauna (omelet, fish, steak) for lunch, then Just Skip Dinner. Human Growth Hormone will be triggered by fasting at night and also by the protein for lunch so the system can auto-perfect. After you eat your fauna and wait about an hour there's a "click" as the system switches into the ketotic state of appetite suppression at which point many people report they can go sixty hours without food or hunger.

"I'll bet eating like this would shrink your stomach and therefore you don't eat as much. Is that the way it is?" KK: That's only part of it. That's the vegan way of looking at things. The truth is animal protein and fat is what makes it a perfectly satisfied lifestyle without any hunger whatsoever. One cannot ever get that satiety with other foods which is why people keep eating. When you eat eat the most calorically dense, not sparse as you're told. Look at foods by their ability to satisfy—the Satiety Index—enabling longer fasting in between which is the real healer.

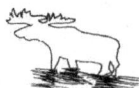

Is coffee or wine bad? KK: They both make me sick with acid but those with strong immunity can enjoy them. When you've had your fill of acid, your body will automatically decline coffee or wine but at other times you'll do just fine. The many pro-wine sites are very convincing so you just have to experiment while always remembering getting drunk is a sin (adversely affecting your kin). It kicked me in the shin so I say "never again": Though it always seemed it would make things better, it never did—so I enjoy the day maximally without this fetter. The sites say one glass for females, two for men—do you really think you can stop at that, my friend? If so, you may give it a go. Regarding coffee, recent studies show that coffee delivers more health benefits than even fruits and vegetables., contributing far more health giving anti-oxidants, and black tea comes second. "Americans get more of their antioxidants from coffee than any other dietary source--nothing else comes close" (Professor Joe Vinson, of Scranton University, Pennsylvania). Whether or not this is true or some coffee addict's self-justifying brew will be up to you. Antioxidants rid the body of free radicals that damage cells and DNA, so this study says coffee drinking reduces risk of liver and colon cancer, type two diabetes. In the past I felt great great with just coffee and cream (and sometimes a little honey in it) I'd have to remember to eat. Coffee drinking and a high fat diet is the best lifestyle, not the worst as we've been taught.

ARTS OF PALEO FASTING

Can you give a recap of the theory please?

FAUNA FIRST AND DAILY FASTING

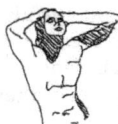

This is written by an ex-fruitarian who found daily fasting after fauna fat to be superior enabling the *inner life*--far superior to all. Man needs fats and nutritionally gut-dense foods of animals to perfectly sustain. The vegan shove-down is plant foods, calorically sparse necessitating all-day eating. The paleo foods are plants, nuts and fauna. "Bliss" is not the Riviera or Vegas, but your own home in the fasting state in which a miraculous new life opens through an inner journey. Daily Fasting is the Key! Higher Paleo Fasting is based on the essentiality of fats which puts the body in fat-burning mode bringing energy and appetite suppression for the daily fast. From fats reverse into short fruit-fasts like the grapecure (raisins), for energy comes from grape carbon. The higher paleo-faster eats occasional fruits and nuts but basically animal. He avoids the vegetables due to anti-nutrients making life hellish.

FAT PHOBIA IS A CULTURAL HYPNOTIC
Stuck in the Rawfoods Movement/Playing Nice

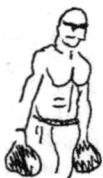

I went with raw vegan fruitarianism for twenty years and made a religion out of it. I didn't achieve mood stability until I ate animal fat (not just avocados). I was constantly hungry (and often angry) so would eat organic rawfood concoctions all day long. As I felt horrible I compensated with superfoods, powders, the whole nine yards. Though visibly declining, I became "orthoexic"--- dogmatically rigid and obsessed with food purity. Despite an initial (short-term) improvement I became miserably isolated and failed to thrive on the long-term. I was so hungry I spent a fortune on these "superfoods" and ate grapes, dates or avocados throughout the day, never feeling satisfied. This movement sounds so good and true but after an early elevation will leave you blue (as seen in the hostile reactions of rawists to any objection to their party line, they haven't a clue). It wasn't until I came back to fauna (animal protein and fat) in the form of raw dairy, eggs and fauna followed by daily fasting that I retrieved total health, svelte and joy because I could now eat once a day only--happy, creative and satisfied. I stayed thin, ageless and stable as food-obsession was finally gone. As beyondveg.com shows, man has always been an omnivore and there've never been true fruitarian

ARTS OF PALEO FASTING

tribes (contrary to raw dogma in both cases). I am so happy eating what my genetic blood calls for.

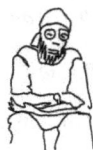

May I include here a study by a paleo anthropologist from University of California: *Karen: Your reversal dieting theory is true from the viewpoint of medical and paleo-anthropology, for early paleo reversals between fat and fruit combined with fasting is confirmed by every study available. Humans are supposed to be lean and healthy as early man sourced high fat meats/marrow, effortlessly transitioned to ketosis and went without food alternating with fruits. This created a unique trigger that stored and then rapidly reduced body fat when reversing between fat-rich or glucose rich foods. As you point out, primitive man having unstable food supplies had to fast, and fat is the only thing making that tenable along with fruits when readily available. I found your site fascinating confirmation of this early evolution. The combo of nuts and dried fruit is so energy dense you can eat far less to be satisfied. Nutritionists argue you need much more variety for essential nutrients but the body's efficiency with daily fasting offsets this need. Without getting anti-oxidants from a lot of fresh fruits and veggies, by fasting (eating little) immunity goes way up, even minimizing the need for anti-oxidants! You apparently have found a strong and massive readership of people who are ready for it. I commend you in your scholarly work and artistic means of presenting it, for it is rock solid. Richard Barnett Ph.D.*

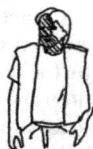

Hunter gatherers who live on very high saturated fat/meat diets are also extremely healthy, lean and vital. Humans perform excellently on paleo foods (meat or fruits) but living on lethal starch combinations damage beta cells and the brain's insulin receptors *so they no longer achieve satiety on minimal quantities of food.* To get this insulin sensitivity back you must eliminate all sweets and starches. The opposite is Raw Till 4: Sugar in the morning and starches in the evening, all you want to prevent hunger feelings. On the long run vegan people are no healthier than anyone else, and suffer from immunity and psychological problems from low protein/fat which causes hormonal imbalances. Bread is used like meat because it is more dense and pushes blood sugar up quickly but gritty for humans, don't give into this. Population growth is destroying our ecosystems and I see the future is grains, grains and more grains: that means more drugs, disease, obesity and lower quality of life, but what can you do? Every time I see my friend nutritionist she is fatter and fatter--it is so insane that people eat 3-5 times a day. All because the foods they eat are so glycemic that they suffer crashes every 3 hours if they don't eat. So sad and unnecessary.

ARTS OF PALEO FASTING

Karen, the Atkins diet actually accelerates protein loss and they lose substantial lean mass even though they are consuming so much protein, so Atkins can never work long term--only your reversal dieting will work! Fasting is referred to as "starvation" dieting in the literature since the Minnesota studies of the 1950's and people are scared to death of missing meals. I also agree with you that some can never return to fruit in any way, they are straight carnivores. Richard Barnett

The prevalent panic over dietary fat is a cultural hypnotic. It makes no sense scientifically once one knows the metabolic processes that follow the eating of fat vs. carbohydrate. We should be a lot more afraid of *being* fat but not at all afraid of dietary fat when eating without carbs. It is very common with vegetarians to substitute over-starch for the deletion of meat and *many vegetarians are still fat.* The consequences of eliminating fat and then gorging on starch and sweet are devastating--never have we had such an obese nation of adults and children!

Question: My idea of fasting is a lot longer period, and why such rigid food routines?

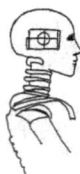

KK: For a super-obese person used to gluttony, eating once a day is a major achievement producing veritable miracles, and it's all about how the brain-body machine works when denying impulses. It's best not to be legalistic with these people, for obesity is everywhere along with family dysfunction, which go together. If you wish to go much longer, go for it! There are plenty of fasting books but this is about a lifelong plan, not just a temporary thing. Fasting is really just a tag line to get to a much deeper theory. In a birdlike engine it's the difference between a good and bad day tomorrow--rigid food routines avoid disaster in a "touchy" high-wired system in which obstructions evoke wild vacillations in mood. I saw during my rawfood phase that too much eating whether good or bad food is the problem. Even with "raw" people are still relying on and thinking too much about FOOD, the biggest device mankind uses to avoid anxiety. (To the same end they're always on freeways and cell phones.) Fasting is bliss--for the right-brain consciousness alone, with the mere *intention* to do it. And just think: we can do it every day! No one ever needs more than one meal a day. If a mother in poverty can scrape together one main meal she need feel no guilt. "Fasting" all depends on where you're at--even Ehret (father of fruitarianism) defined it as "just eating less". Just one meal skipped evokes the fasting process: fasting consciousness and positive healing forces (PHF). In fact, the mere intention to fast evokes that wonderful spirit. For some eating

ARTS OF PALEO FASTING

three meals a day, just skipping 7 lunches a week--Ramadan Fasting--can eliminate old obstructions and habits. It's amazing how just one new habit can transform your life forever. The bible gives various types of fasts: some are no sugar, some no meat, etc. It all depends where you start--just by not doing what you're usually doing (to avoid anxiety) you can reprogram the brain--what we call transformation of energy or "making gold".

I saw that just about all my bad habits were mal-adaptive coping devices while living in civilization. But, alone in nature, man clears! When no more identity-smears, no more tears. Then in purity out goes the fears and we open up to new careers. I hate legalism when it comes to fasting, for it cuts out 90% of the human race from ever trying it. Just skipping dinner every day so that human growth hormone--which comes out at night with fasting--can perfect and youthify the engine is a major achievement of a few . Once one sees the efficacy of just one meal missed, he begins to enjoy fasting and will attempt longer and longer fasts--that's up to him, not legalistic dogma as to what constitutes the "true fast".

Question: There are some schools of thought, though I am skeptical, that believe that whereas not eating at all is relatively safe for most people, but that eating only a little (less than 1000 calories for men, 800 calories for women) can be unsafe as it is not good for internal organs.

KK: The whole world is so hungry so it can't imagine fat-fasting. One reader said "one piece of pizza and I have to spend the whole next day on a tread mill". They've got things so wrong—just have as much melted cheese as you want—without starch—and then enjoy your fasting day. These present theories you speak of are not taking the pleasant (appetite-suppressing and fat-burning) properties of fat into account. Whatever this theory is, it isn't about fat-fasting. I tell you truly, I can eat one-half chicken breast in the morning and not hungry until the next morning. This theory says fasting evokes HGH and ketosis putting one in hunger-free health, whereas eating little might not trigger HGH since the reserves aren't depleted. Fast 22 hours and stay bone thin and energetic from early in the morning until late at night, when all wrongs are made right with fasting (going light). Moreover, in the summer we eat fruit too and we're still the same bone-thin in view.

Question: of course, eating less than 1000 calories for someone who is underweight is dangerous.

ARTS OF PALEO FASTING

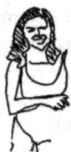

KK But think on this: Many skinny or anorexic aren't assimilating-- and thus fasting is the same prescription to increase assimilation and thus healthy weight. Many skinny show scrawny arms and legs--a mass of wrinkles, because though skinny they are nevertheless obstructed on a cellular level and can't assimilate nor eliminate the mucus at the base of each wrinkle. A day fast brings recession of this mucus level as the "mass of wrinkles" smooth out to clear perfection. People are shocked to hear that the ultra-skinny or anorexics would be fasted in order to gain healthy tissue.

Question: One thing is becoming clear -- the high occurrence of food allergies for people -- so it is good for people with arthritis, headaches, etc to consult with a doctor about a rotation diet where single food is consumed more than once within a 5 to 7 day period. Please respond.

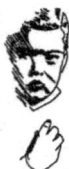

KK: The increased allergy (as well as all other diseases) problem comes from immuno-suppression. Daily fasting after animal fat (tiny potent) strengthens immunity more than any other method. After longterm failed veganism one is so immuno-suppressed they can't eat anything. Find *one* thing even if caviar and you'll begin to accept other, and then all foods again. Among other things protein enhances immunity while refined starches suppress it. How interesting that this is happening in this New Age vegan era as increasingly the whole world is going vegan assuming it's healthier--but a suppressed immune system isn't healthy and thus the increased incidence of allergies, mood problems, and MCS—Multiple Chemical Sensitivities. Suppressed immunity promotes obesity since the system doesn't detox as well. Just look at people in the fifties--they ate far more animal protein and fat and stayed thin, energetic, and stable compared to the bloat, mood swings and depression of today.

Question: Such a fast can be extended by intake of fat -- good fat -- such as natural walnut oil, organic olive oil, Haines All Blend Oil or other high grade vegetable oil, etc.

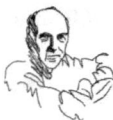

KK The vegan era overestimates the importance of fruit, nut and fractured vegetable fats while discounting the efficacy (while vilifying) animal fats--fauna. Some of them, incredibly, even think vegetable fats are ok (because they "sound" ok) though their link to cancer is evident. Whether we like it or not (or whether we love animals or not) man has adapted to eating animal fat from the beginning

ARTS OF PALEO FASTING

(beyondveg.com). These poor misled vegans look old earlier because they don't eat animal fat. Paleo enthusiasts are shining handsome specimens of the race. Vegetable fats cooked at high temperatures can kill you--those are the killers, not the animal fat—as everything is backwards and "all popular notions are false". And I doubt anyone could live on olive oil but one could live on cheese. Animal fat is substantive, and only small amounts are needed for long periods of satiation and fasting.

Question: As for changing habits and routines, this is always good -- one should mix it up -- this is what separates us from machines. When one follows the same routine without change daily there is the risk of shifting over to automatic and not fully participating in the joy of eating/assimilating.

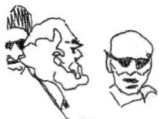

KK: This is another very common fallacy (that man is a multivariate) because city life promotes variety. Primitive man living in one area often had the same mono diet for his entire life. But if one is living in wilderness solitude, survival depends on routines, and buying bulk simplifies all supplies for the household: a short list, but great quantity of each. For the fastarian recluse the unchanging food life sounds monotonous but remember in fastarian consciousness it is no longer the food that matters, except insofar as it fuels and suppresses appetite for the day's activities and the most intense sensory adventure. Boring? No—because as interest in food variety lessens, experience and perceptual acuity increases, as through fasting he achieves experience. The fastarian embarks on a proprioceptive journey from which there is no return: Encased in monotony, the inner life flourishes into greatest creative variety. Remember, most people eat for entertainment--their interest is in the food and eating. For the fastarian, eating isn't the entertainment--it's the consciousness afterwards! In this situation, less is definitely more.

Comment: Musically, this translates to exploring a wide variety of music because you're holding one thing constant.

KK: Definitely--variety keeps the brain shifting. It is interesting how people listen to the same music identified to their group but never explore their own inner realm. Feeling good once more, you go inside.

Question: We are designed to be able to handle periods of food scarcity, so is it not best to make food scarce in one's life every once and a while and for some people, even for extended periods?

ARTS OF PALEO FASTING

KK That's a very interesting thought--Some may even be at their best when fasting, as if they were born to stretch their survival skills as the biggest part of their destiny.

Question: I agree that highly heated vegetable oils are not healthy. And then vegetables fried in such oils, particularly potatoes, are pretty risky food sources if regularly eaten. Certainly having French fried potatoes several times a weak is not very wise.

KK Even if using olive oil it wrecks my system for weeks--that's the hypersensitive: transgressing rigid food restrictions obstructs happy regular routines. The Indians fry potatoes in olive oil and curry--I could never take that. Starch and fat do not mix.

Question: Can you elaborate on why you think the fruitarian diet is no good? I guess if one tried to duplicate a natural diet it would be rich in fruits (particularly berries), nuts, roots, lice and termites. I suspect primitive man ate lots of bugs--a good source of protein and low in cholesterol. The fruitarian diet assumes that natural is best but then neglects to encourage the eating of bugs. In addition, I suspect primitive humans also had fish, birds, shellfish and even rodents and other small mammals when he could. None of this cooked, of course.

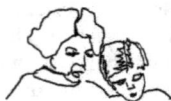

KK I may have fruits in summer season but basically it confuses the system. Just a chicken breast or two in the morning and I'm good for all-day workin'. You don't need bugs or rodents—you need clean animal foods which you can easily procure, and just a little suits for the day. This is how you bring up kids: with good food and plenty of ray. Yes, the paleo diet (2.3 million years) is fruit, vegetables, meat, nuts and berries. The starchy modern diet is only 10,000 years old--not enough time for humans to adapt/the nutrients are crap. We are only truly adapted to the paleo diet of 5 categories of food. The fruitarian dogma says "apes were fruitarian"—not true. Apes eat fruits and bugs (carnivore). They also say "Garden of Eden man was fruitarian" but never has there been paleo-evidence of any fruitarian tribe on the earth--they all had some animal protein. We can call any animal source--bugs or body--as FAUNA. Man needs fauna just like the cat--that means animal fat. Cats and humans have the exact same needs (this is opposite to all the fat-phobic food dogma of today, which is why many are fat). Animal fat burns fat off the body, due to the effects of glucagons vs. insulin. After 20 years of "fruitarianism" I regained health by easing into a cheese omelet each morning (fauna fat) followed by fasting all day and with any fruit just a fig at night (rarely, I didn't need it). Fruitarianism as well as vegan diets bring a "failure to thrive" and circuitous mental logic preventing recovery which only comes from eating animal products. I love animals too, but will never sacrifice my health on the altar of health dogma again.

Question: Processed foods are indeed a problem and not so prevalent in the 1950's as they are now. And the bulk of the processed food chosen to replace animal foods (including snake oil superfoods snacks) is grain or vegetable based – sugar, cookies, crackers, twinkies, cupcakes, donuts, potato chips, tortilla chips, etc. Speak please

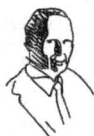

KK The public is mis-led from "medical consensus panels" who themselves fear malpractice and are simply caving into vegan "raw" pressure. It's happening in media, schools and even churches who feel more holy from the vegan diet (false, the bible never said it). The befuddled public thinks this crap is safer than animal fat/dreaded cholesterol. Actually, fat burns cholesterol off the body but beyond that we *desperately need cholesterol* which forms the brain, the synapses and all the insulated wirings. It is insulin which cues the liver to create it's own cholesterol--insulin created from starch. If we just eat animal fat, all cholesterol is burned out. Shame on the AMA for not telling us this: Cancer and heart disease was rare before 1920---when coca cola (sugar) and refined flour mills began. That's when the heart attacks and cancer started: insulin brings the cell proliferation called cancer and prevents cholesterol from being burned off. The problem is this: There are only three macronutrients: protein, fat and carbohydrate. If in fear (cultural fat-phobia) we eliminate fat, we also eliminate protein (since they go together). We must substitute with something--and carb is all that is left. Ergo, the vegan is getting way too much starch, and no fauna. Paleo macronutrient ratios (of healthy aborigines) is something like 65% protein and fat, and 35% carbohydrate in the form of fruits, veggies, nuts, berries, roots etc. Compare that to the modern vegan-inspired diet of 75% carbohydrate and little fauna and you see an unbelievable difference. Thus, humans don't look human anymore. Look in National Geographic magazines from the fifties--people looked great and fit. The women were slim like Harriet Nelson and the men looked like Paul Newman. But now, never have we seen such bulky and distorted specimens! Man (the hunter) is supposed to look elegant, svelte, tall and thin with an enlarged brain (called encephalization). Paleo man had strong bones and teeth. Starchy vegan man (the farmer) is short and dumb (de-encephalized brain) with brittle bones, fat, and crumbled teeth--like the ancient Egyptians. They were not svelte like the images painted on their walls--they were filled with fat, dental decay and every modern degenerative disease because of their farmer diet resembling our modern vegan diet: fruits, veggies, starches, honey, and a little meat. Does this not sound exactly like what you'd read in *Cosmopolitan*? Think of all the wives killing their poor husbands with the wrong food--all the while thinking they're doing good. For complete information on this discrepancy between paleo science (high fat is high tech) and modern (low-fat) food dogma read my *Champion Guides.*

Question: Many may choose sea bugs like lobster and crab over land animals like beef. Currently, I eat fish a couple times a week, shrimp once a week (a type of bug) and splurge on clams (bug/mollusk), oysters (bug/mollusk), scallops (bug/mollusk), crab (bug), lobster (bug).

KK: Scavengers, disgusting but enjoy em! Though the sea bugs are unclean (like catfish) meant to suck up bacteria from the earth (like the pig), put that aside when you imbibe--I know they are delicious like all scavengers and it's just another paradox that unclean things taste best to humans .

Question: Now, with all the pollutants, this might be something worth thinking about, but I suspect that the lower in the food chain you go the safer it is since this stuff accumulates in fat and muscle tissue -- so may not be great to eat a scavenger, but even worse to eat the animals that eat the scavengers.

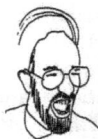

KK: We don't eat carnivores like dogs but pigs are herbivores by nature just like deer and cows. The Muslims copied kosher, having admired the Jews for all their regulations so they called their aversion to pig *halal* but it's got nothing to do with science or religion. They copied the Jews and went extreme.

Question: Same with cats and dogs -- not sure why they are unclean, but would guess there is an explanation.

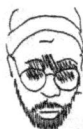

KK Dogs are carnivores basically, although vegan owners make em eat veggies, fruits or sickening dog food they'd much rather have raw meat. Camels are the last to be slaughtered in times of famine then people's pets: cats and dogs which are man's best friends—it's unbelievable how they can't see the emotions of these animals who respond to humans. They must be differentiated from other animals used for food—the fact that they aren't is a reflection of the New Age society which *homogenizes* everything into the same level—a cockroach, a dog, a human all the same. In the old days man's best friend had Special Status but liberals hate that, especially the vegans, so uncool.

Question: I was vegan 12 years and I can't believe I'm eating meat. I feel so much better though and my life has taken off, relieved of this burden plus all the endless food preparations.

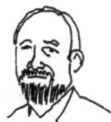

KK You now have Found Time to accomplish everything you ever wanted. The addicted food life consumes all your time like any drug used to escape (your supposed fate) but now you'll see you were destined to be great.

ML: I like what you say about keeping a clean house and it is a mystery to me why people don't keep their homes clean as they lower their quality of life in many ways by having a dirty house.

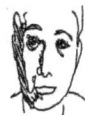

KK It is worse than disgusting, a product of feminism. Don't complain of your cold husbands when your homes resemble a pigsty. Love your spouse and family—fix longcooking pot roasts they smell for hours, that's a happy house. A man will cherish a female if she maintains a nice home for him but now women are above being consigned to housework and maintaining order, for this is a job that is literally never done. They want to copy the male world of many projects hastily accomplished rather than the female role of constant work for a happy home. But if they don't continuously establish order, the place is a mess not a happy and spiritually elevating environment. To keep a creative atmosphere which evokes thought and cheer it must be one's first priority but now women are too busy outside the home in work, play or "cruising". Is it any wonder men leave slovenly feminist wives at a rate of 6/10? When I broach this subject I am banned from the list if it's filled with feminists.

Question: Well, I don't see this cleanliness topic as gender related -- responsible people of either sex have an obligation to keep their areas clean and themselves clean.

KK Yes, that's true. But in a marriage it's a matter of the division of labor. I'm happy to keep house if my husband takes care of the electronics, the business, the plumbing and keeps the cars going.

Leave Veggies for Rabbits

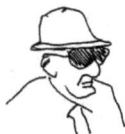

Eat em and get Sick from Anti-Nutrients

Many of you due to insulin resistance depend on veggies and non-sweet fruits like tomatoes, red bells and squash because you can't take sugar. The damaged metabolism through veganism can't tolerate cooked or raw vegetables without adverse results—feeling big and sluggish. Eat meat and it melts right in, gut stays flat, you're high as a kite day and night. We know the type of food eaten determines morphology—size and shape. Below is the dialogue between two experimenters who ate veggies after a long term higher paleo-fasting diet. They were both supremely healthy--one from fauna-fasting and the other a lacto-fruitarian diet, but both witnessed a radical decline with damp, limp, soggy vegetables (raw or cooked).

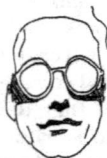

We happy fatarians (slick and thin) experimented with vegetables for three days and both got sick, bloating up like couches. It was a terrible experience and our entire disposition changed. We always saw veggies as innocent and healthy yet the reaction was worse than with fauna. If fauna is the only thing you don't react to, you're a universal reactor (an obligate fauna-faster) and veggies could kill you! Children are very right to hate vegetables. If you are meant to live on fruit or pure fauna and nothing else, all other foods will be sadly inferiorizing--it is the Lion's or Eagle's Diet. The following is the transcript of our common experiment with vegetables. One experimenter was a pure faunivore, the other optimized on fruits, nuts and dairy.

Dialogue Between Two Sick Experimenters:

Larry: Ever since eating these cooked vegetables I have bloated legs (like tree trunks--very painful) and several other allergic reactions--a real "thud" in consciousness--bleakness, depression, cynicism--a very definite downturn!

ARTS OF PALEO FASTING

Jerry: We both had the same reaction: Whereas meat melts right in, the most digestible of all foods, I had asparagus with tummy upsets, spaciness, swollen eyes and have been bloated the whole day, same with cauliflower. I am back to the Lion Diet--high paleo for good.

Larry: I ate asparagus before noon and I am still bloated. I will need 24 hours to wash this out of my system. If I don't feel better by tomorrow I will fast. I feel like 200 pounds, and groggy.

Jerry: Right--vegetables are for the other animals--rabbits, etc. Yuk! Never have I felt this lousy--puffy, down, depressed.

Larry: I am going to sell my canned asparagus for a penny for a can. I am laughing but I bought a whole bunch the other day. Little did I know I was digging my grave! But it is important to experiment.

Jerry: I do the same--overbuy when I get on a tangent (indicating addiction-food?) and am always so glad to get back to "reality"--the straight and narrow, the best and most delicious—a freezer full of meats.

Larry: Yep, I get excited and buy food in large quantities, anticipating the feast cuz I'm famished from not eating meat. That made me a food addict but now I see veganism did it.

Jerry: I bought frozen string beans today--wonder if they'll be the same way. Terrible--it had been years since I'd had veggies and now I know why. They're always reinforced with starch in a meal, no wonder the human race is bloated and fat.

Larry: Can you imagine people eating these veggies with potatoes or noodles—stuffing. How are they functioning? I want a nice steak to propel me for two days not these silly veggies.

Jerry: Isn't it funny that fauna doesn't effect us this way--supposedly the most hazardous; and yet vegetables--what the world calls innocent bloats us up like couches?

Larry: It is amazing. I have eaten Red Salad {tomato, red bell} and never felt awful like after asparagus. If there's any bloat with non-sweet red fruit salad it's gone in one hour--not like this veggie hangover.

ARTS OF PALEO FASTING

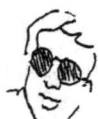

Jerry:: The spittum tastes so bitter--the damp soggy vegetables bog the body down trying to digest them. They were meant for other animals but man in his ego thinks everything is for him to eat, just like the oats for the horses. I just had some chicken and feel immeasurably better.

Larry: I want to know more about fauna fasting--like a lovely lioness, very independent, regal and living on meat and fat--creating one's own kingdom free of vegetables!

Jerry: Think I'll throw them out to the rabbits--or would that be cruel? Because just look at humanity--they don't look in the image of God and most of them are very sick, all involved with doctors. And it affects their mood! I feel absolutely sick but a good nights rest will bring recovery.

Larry: I used to eat oats. I even was eating them raw thinking they were healthy.

Jerry: Horrors--you didn't realize they're for horses? Hey I know what we can do with the oats--boil them in water then smother it with milk and honey and eat it for breakfast! hah. It's like the "stuffers of starch" thinking they're doing a good thing, all because grains are low in calories.

Larry: Starch-eaters who worship their doctors are like fossils to me. I can't relate to the "follower" mentality anyway.

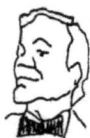

Jerry: They get roped in to Big Pharma and tests and the whole profession who encourages that kind of eating. It is simply tragic--people moving out of the desert they love, just to be "close to their doctors", all the while eating like pigs--or better put, rabbits. It's that same doctors who deny rampant candida.

Larry: It's a major theoretical change: veggies aren't just secondary, they're crap! I once heard this from a health food store owner--that greens were poison carcinogens--everyone called him crazy of course.

Larry:: By the way, oddly enough, I got myself to feel better last night by eating cheese. Go figure! I had a small piece of cheddar and felt so much better. Weird?

ARTS OF PALEO FASTING

Jerry: Just increased immunity--your body is saying "thanks for ceasing the rabbit food--I'll now reward you with dairy and a stable belly, your birthright as a human being."

Larry:: I like how you mention the children's instinctual revulsion against vegetables.

Jerry:: Right--just think how they're forced to sit there until they eat it. Is it any wonder they turn to sweet starches and fast food, just to escape?

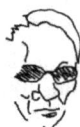

Larry: *The Zone* diet says to eat tons of veggies and I can't think of a book that says to avoid them. What happened in Atkins was the low fat fakes buzzed in with veggies, salads and "Atkins Low Fat" then kidney disease--no way for organs to clean out toxicity without fat.

Jerry: So true--I was thrown off an Atkins list for putting UP fat and UP fasting. They wanted low fat meats--they just couldn't "get it".

Larry: The only veggies I can handle are occasional leaves when I go out to watch others pig out on the most preposterous things and yet these same people ridicule me for drinking coffee.

Jerry: Yes, fruitarian species like apes also eat leaves--these are different from eating plants. And coffee is actually a cleanser, as fast as a grape, with more antioxidants than produce. Coffee houses were always for the intellectuals.

Larry: Oh I didn't realize that leaves are different than plants--so occasional romaine should be ok then.

Jerry: Absolutely--all fruitarian species eat leaves (not filled with anti-nutrients) but not necessarily plants. Man is made to enjoy juicy fruit--but do you necessarily have a craving for raw broccoli? Yuk! Would a child want raw broccoli, or some grapes or pizza?

Larry: That cheddar is so good. I gave in last night to recover from the veggies. I broke out the Little Dipper, warmed it with olive oil. It was greasy heavenly messing bliss! Ha!

Jerry: Oh yes, absolutely--very soothing. The greasier the better the elimination. My neighbor refused to give his dog gravy (which he craved) because it brought on diarrhea! I say good! That poor fat vegan dog needed to eliminate.

EPILOGUE

Do you have a natural craving for raw broccoli or cauliflower? Tell the truth—it's not there. Salads without greasy dressing? Rare. Man craves fats, animal fats, and no plant fat like avocado will take care of that. I crave fruit for refreshment and meat for satiety and re-invigoration. And if I can't stand the sugar, water will do.

I am amazed and overjoyed that all I need is 1-2 breasts and that's it for the day. What could be more efficient than that? After all that all-day eating and never being satisfied, always looking for more, then buying a wealth of superfoods to compensate which just made me sick—I gotta tell the world about this!

After decades of worthless plant eating we moved to our new home. I don't know why, but suddenly I didn't know what to eat. Nothing made sense to me, there was no logic to anything, I was just flailing around. Just to fill up I ate starches, then to feel legit with the raw crowd I had banana smoothies. Lost, billious, unhappy.

When I switched to meat, *suddenly* my food life made sense. Only meat "lighted up" in my perception, it alone had meaning. And the biggest meaning was NO MORE EATING: a day of just creativity.

Forget the debunked China Study or MacDougal who says since all continents have existed on starch, that must mean it's right or max. Man lives 1/12 his normal lifespan from the Garden of Eden and he's getting sicker/gotten much fatter and his brain is mush accepting the narrative of new age chatter.

You *can* live on starches but life won't be what it promises to be: Happy and comfy in your home with a pot roast cooking and family gathered around. Until you enjoy that rebound after fruitarianism you won't know what that great traditional homey life means I've found.

P.S. This book is not for raw meat enthusiasts but those enjoying the aroma of pot roast for several hours in the home. It's our tradition: American family bonding.

Study of a Cerebrotonic Introvert Overcomer

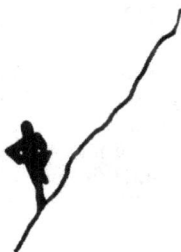

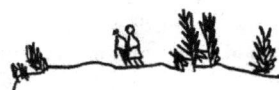

The young child never disappears but other layers are superimposed on its core. Deep inside the baby's still the same but the *forces acted on it*--the twists and turns all determine the shapes it assumes. If that center be a bottomless hole it's filled with reckless extravagance or prodigious idiosyncrasies which get worse with age but with repentance and God's help this all transforms to monastic reclusion, extremely high boundaries and creative bliss!

She came from a famous family of evangelists, popular orators and writers in Scotland all Calvinist Scholars. Among a long lineage of ancestors sharing the same gifts her uncle was David MacLennan, a mega-church leader who wrote 20 books on homiletics with a lifelong tenure at Yale. Fired with the same enthusiasm for psychology, theology and theories she followed the same tradition of prolific output but with deep and archetypal illustrations and a formula which defines a True Theory in the Life Sciences (Koestler 1962) Her story was a very hard road starting out as a toad but ending in one of the best stories ever told.

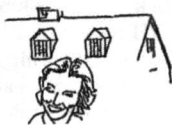

Introvert. As a child she was always alone and involved in projects, hobbies and lessons. It was a busy but solitary childhood complicated with alcoholism in the home where God was rarely mentioned and religion remained watered down and indifferent. As early as puberty she had a thirst

ARTS OF PALEO FASTING

for God, a desire to ascend to another reality beyond the world. She had problems entering school at 5 as "school phobia" combined with the fear of coming home.

GOING INSIDE

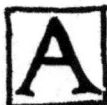

A The introvert adapted to the fears of her world by "going inside" to another reality as a straight A student. Her parents being quite elderly and her two older sisters away at college she was basically an only child but felt envy, hostility and triangulation from the sisters—and this sense of being disliked and out of place formed the early template of her life. "It was always two against one. It hurt being the subject of gossip and gang-ups but that's how it is in primitive life before you learn how to adapt and stay intact—for to this thorny situation, I surely did react." A fearful misfit status created a sense of rejection and discontinuity with her whole generation, resulting in an inward solitary life in which she became quite well developed in painting, drawing, music and detailed projects (e.g. like learning all the names and positions of bones and muscles in the human body by age 9). She dealt with outer chaos by immersion and extreme dedication to her own inner life which meant she was totally alone until the end.

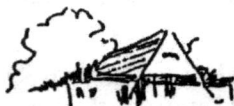

Recluse. As a teen in the sixties moral relativism was taught in the public schools, teaching there were no moral absolutes. "What is bad for one is good for another—so anything goes." She was told not to judge anything as "bad" and even the word "moral" or "sin" brought social rebuff. The result was that despite early talents and academic success her life became unstable for two decades. She worked hard with straight A's but got drunk at night. This was compounded by her alcoholic mother--she was terrified of her and her father also alcoholic was too docile to defend her. Though they both stopped drinking before they died and she later learned to appreciate their good qualities, collateral damage of alcoholism along with sibling hostilities dug deep templates. All these fears left when she became mom's drinking buddy at age 16—it was like a ton of bricks fell off her shoulders. "Alcohol answered all my childhood problems." However, with outer society she lacked boundaries and felt degraded and invaded with which she coped through addictions of all kinds. It was the sixties and moral breakdown was creating insanity, ruin, poverty and divorce but it would take decades to see the horrid results. America was witnessing a barbaric invasion

ARTS OF PALEO FASTING

from within and no one could tell baby boomers what was right or wrong—
they would live the way they wanted with no respect for authority.

OFF TO SCHOOL

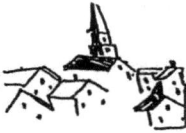

Having been sheltered in an alcoholic environment she
was a misfit in society. Her life was split between
academic excellence and solitary creative pursuits but the
major interest was Family Systems Theory--how the
family as a system keeps one person down--the
"identified" patient--and this absorbed the rest of her
formal education. "I was peculiarly fitted for this study because of my early
family situation."

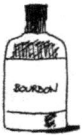

Of particular interest was the Wife of the Alcoholic Syndrome." Here
the wife is constantly complaining about her husband's drinking but
when he finally gets sober she tries to trip him up. "That is systems
theory: the family system adapts to the problem which becomes the
status quo, its level of homeostasis. Recovery is too much of a change
and the family cannot adapt." She wrote her doctoral thesis on the
psychology of neurotic interaction (A System's Theoretic View of Pathologic
Interaction) on sick systems surrounding all disease—alcoholism, overeating,
psychosis, anorexia.

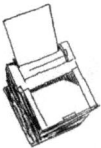

The huge dissertation was acclaimed "rings a bell, filled with poetic
cadence and nail-hitting-on-the-head alliterations that make for
fascinating evocative reading" (UCI). She developed her own style
of Johannesse Verse by advancing a theory of human nature
delivered in machine-gun style using alliterations and examples
drawn from nature and mythology. A good start but there was
much to learn before it could be brought before the public. Despite popular
pleas to make it a book her interests continued to expand and "timing was
wrong. I had yet to go through three decades of hell to get a hard shell and get
ready to yell—I became a lady *after* I fell".

ARTS OF PALEO FASTING

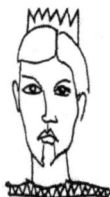

For three years she wrote about the systems surrounding all diseases especially alcoholism and anorexia, culminating in a huge grant-funded manuscript called The Contagion of Madness. But being still undifferentiated from the original family system she caved into mental illness and going home on weekends. "The med profession had me on anti-depressants which miscombined with alcohol".

NEW PSYCHOLOGY BASED ON ENERGY

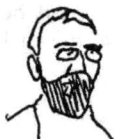

After many silent years she began to build back up. Now her theories burgeoned into a new matrix on par with Freud and Jung. Her interests in pathological systems began to include "most social behavior as approval-seeking in the pecking-order. It's all just negotiation of meaning and consensual validation--not true reality." To this budding social theorist mundane reality was beginning to look absurd: "Yak-yak-yak saying nothing while talking all the time. Whether church or coffee-klatch the social arena seemed petty, mean, boring and shallow." This perception of culture began to dominate her writing--"not focusing on evident pathology but seeing just about everything as pathological. I had outgrown the university and was tired of talking about the system of pathology--I wanted to take on culture at large." "The Book"--her life's work--was not due to culminate for twenty more "fateful fretful years" of painful learning experiences in human systems theory. "I wrote constantly in my journal to overcome current crises but it was only to grow. There were more labor pains before giving birth."

HIGH AS THE SKY PHASE

At this point her life changed completely splitting from culture and family and taking on a different name "Maria Civetta." All of her artistic talents from youth re-surfaced by exploring other cultures. "I transcended American culture and everything I knew and became joyous and enraptured as I was thrust into new worlds and untapped reservoirs of creativity inside." She moved to San Diego and bought a "condominium in the sky" turning it into an Italian Villa with mirrors and tiles from floor to ceiling throughout. It was a magnificent palace on the ninth floor overlooking Balboa Park and was put in a full-page spread in San Diego Magazine (1980) entitled "Villa Design." "I was on top of the world." It was there she met her husband for the next five years.

In Her Own Words on the Ontologically Fatal Insight that Life Isn't What You Thought It was:

"I wanted to do so many things artistically and academically with many avenues yet to explore. I soared to the heights but would recurrently relapse into just thinking--or even drinking." But then in 1981 sitting atop her villa in the sky the entire theory applying Einstein's field theory to psychology came out. As the basis of this new view was the formula: all disease obstruction, all recovery elimination, all success attraction. This was to be the matrix for *Champion Guides* and *Manual for Superior Men* in ten books decades later.

DOWN IN THE DUMPS WITH THE CHUMPS

She remained true to her solitary inner life and this meant going bankrupt. "How could I make money in isolation? I was only happy in withering solitude." Her writings said "insulate-detach and develop your own inner reality an inner journey of enlightenment. The outer is a mere wasted life." How true this turned out to be for soon the 'real learning' occurred-"my Ph.D. in the streets." She went bankrupt as her work was "still in scattered forces-- I wasn't ready and still very immature." She lost her villa in the sky and had to move back home. The return to the original family system "was psychotic shock and the ontologically fatal insight that the world was not what I thought it was." She had felt terror as her whole reality collapsed. "I had changed so much since leaving home ten years earlier and now was confronted with the original system and all of its prejudices. I felt just like a Jew in Nazi Germany and the collision was catastrophic. My siblings absorbed my older husband into their system and the whole thing came down on me hard."

CINDERELLA AND A DRUNKEN FELLA

"My husband usually sober and adoring started drinking and in joining their ranks became rank. In fear I became a collapsed shack lost in despair and hopelessness." All of her "high as the sky" hopes were dashed and she became a "sickly captive, a nothing. The most likely to succeed became a has-been-who-never-was, an invalid locked in the smallest room in the house." Having lost independence the sisters and husband gained total control just as her parents began to recede and die. "My only protection was gone--it was now totally a conspiratorial climate." Her previous life of happy optimism and freedom broke down as an incredible dream to be replaced by great tribulation, a psychic nightmare lasting two decades. "I was terrified of my liberal feminist older sisters so coldly different from me with no understanding or respect. I was treated like a thing, an illness to which I mal-adapted through alcoholic relapses. The wages of sin is death—even though I drank in reaction, the results are still psychological death and network disgust. The biggest mal-adaptation of the wife of the alcoholic is slipping into alcoholism herself. If we don't learn how to adapt to sick situations without becoming sick we face the same ramifications. Whenever I would talk of my future plans like writing books they would threaten to institutionalize me for my 'delusions of grandeur.' This was a scary era perfect for a horror movie and I thank God every single day for saving me from it."

When weak elements get power they abuse it. In Greek family tragedies like the 'three sisters' (two against one) childhood rivalries are magnified into adult life: All is blamed on the "odd girl out" and anything positive is re-labeled as negative by the secret alliance of the two. Adapting to Greek tragedy nuances opened up whole areas of study as these episodes became fodder for chapters like "Anorexic Systems" "Bad Faith or Fullness?" and especially "Fallen Hero Syndrome". Her life was a caricature for the vicissitudes of many a writer's life: being up, falling down and rebuilding back up again. As she got weaker in this system--despite having written about systems theory and supported by grants to do so--the result was psychotic fear, crippling low self-esteem and loss of identity. Her sisters became "meaner", her husband "drunker" until in 1985 her father died, the marriage was annulled and she exiled to the desert.

A BROKEN POT SAVED

She who was voted the most likely to succeed was a broken pot shattered to pieces. But life was now going to build back up for it was just in this hostile environment and morose phase that she came to God through Jesus Christ. " I learned the most important thing: Christ said 'They hated me before they hated you—they love only their own, the others they despise. Have fear if all men think well of you, friendship with the world is enmity with God.'" She learned to expect tribulation, and to see the *bondage* of sin--the very sins the culture now condoned. The family--meant to be a loving fortress in an evil world--was breaking down all around. Plastic people filled with projections-- harrowing harassing harridans without a heart and calling it 'tough love.' I saw everything about human nature in a new light especially in the Psalms. Feminism made many meaner than men."

In this period she became quite cynical about the ungodly in both sexes: " Men were bad but women were worse. While men were hostile and aggressive the feminist influence made women jealous and untrustworthy." So the ambitious female ended up working alone in silence. She saw the nineties as the era when "inferior men ruled while the superior were stuck in the periphery. To conform to the group was 'moral' and to stand apart was 'immoral.' I found so much solace in the Bible which continuously speaks of persecution and the cross had major significance for me: the atonement was complete and I was free--of past people and paltry sins. I could now just enjoy the magic moment." Thus began her detachment from the outer to venture deep into the inner. She saw how "the nobles walked on foot while the idiots and thieves rode horseback." All of this was fodder for her books to frustrated fallen (heroes) of the future: *Manual for Superior Men* and *Champion Guides.*

TO THE HAPPY DESERT WE GO

It was then that she "left civilization entirely" for a cabin in the desert wilderness ten miles out of a small desert town. She embarked on an inner journey with God: "sweet solitude, precious privacy--the outer world was finally gone. The further I got from people and their social expectations the happier I got." Not religion but relationship with God was what she wanted now. "Not a horizontal relationship to people (churchists and groupies) but a vertical one with the Creator of it all. I found my destiny as female home-maker in a small cabin on 230 acres with dogs and cats." It was here walking all day in the wilderness and riding a bike that she found the unique blueprint of her life. From a watered-down and indifferent religion in youth came a full-blown reality of the divine--surrounded by animals, angels and the spiritual writings of evangelist-ancestors from her Scottish roots. My whole conception of family and heritage changed. I was so surprised and delighted to have woken up to the blood in my veins while transcending the people problems in *this* life."

CHURCH BESMIRCHED SHE SEARCHED

She thought if she joined a church she could relate to like-minded people but instead felt out of place, maligned, gossiped about, sided against and misjudged. "I saw churchists as Pharisees--there was no real devotion here just the blind habit of church attendance. These types were the worst for this caste-like social conformity is the opposite to Christianity. I wanted only The Word, silence, contemplation, meditation, prayer and fasting. I didn't want this social hall religion and their petty pot-lucks. I refused to partake in silly conversations where the trivial was mixed with the important--'social hebephrenia" or 'word salad': jocularity, chattering, forced hilarity, logorrhea and constant jesting. They rarely spoke of God just people. I wanted just to be alone in nature as a Christian Mystic. No more religion, groups or hierarchies--just relationship with the Master—"my loving Creator who had been through the same scapegoat system while here on earth. Who else could speak to my lonely misunderstood misfit status?"

ALONE AT LAST

"Alone in nature, man clears." When finally free of society suddenly all her art background came out in 5000 drawings which became the basis for the Champion Guides Karen Kellock PictureStrips. She was so artistically prolific in this period that 900 pages of picture strips poured out in two years. The entire picture-strip is--"neurophysiologically speaking--far superior to text-only for evoking mass insight. Words and images are dynamite--a thousand times more powerful as a psychological medium on a world scale."

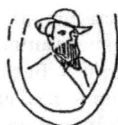

It was then she became acquainted with her famous evangelist and writer-ancestors in Scotland. "They were great Calvinists, which is how America began. It was the opposite to the Armenian error we see today in most all churches and televangelists. In total solitude I explored Calvinism in great depth and woke-up to the blood in my veins. My uncle was David MacLennan, a famous author and mega-church leader. He wrote 20 books with much the same theories, yet we never met. I also read my grandfather and great-grandfather's writings and couldn't believe the similarities of thoughts which were genetic. What great joy I had, *a family at last*--this was the genetic clan. After so many tragic years mal-adapting to relations with no relation, now I walked tall."

ISOLATION: INDIAN DESIGNS

Flourishing in her home life "I had arrived. Home is all--home is where it's at. If only modern women can see this. Home is where a female can detach and develop her own inner reality, an inner journey of enlightenment. The outer is

ARTS OF PALEO FASTING

a mere wasted life. Feminism had torn down my home--where I belong, where I do my best work. Home is the only protection for females, as the gifted element in a cruel world! My home is my rock, fortress and castle. And so insofar as feminists tear it down I guess that makes me anti-feminist. The feminists trivialized housework so now many homes look like a bomb hit them. I feel sorry for their poor children and husbands surrounded by dirty disorder and a disheveled wife and mother--who demands respect while not commanding it."

Encamped in her cozy cabin "another spirit came over me. Everything flourished through Indian Designs on clothes and walls as esoteric world music filled the rooms. Again I was coming into a separate reality from the mass. As an artist I adventurously allowed myself these new avenues. As I left the West an interest in fasting came center to my life and I investigated Ramadan. Without knowing it since the age of 16 I was already doing it: eating one predawn meal then enjoying the day in energetic activity, prayer and contemplation and a real sense of accomplishment at night." She soon saw daily mini-fasting as crucial to championship-- an entirely new view of fasting simply done while getting all benefits thereof. "It was the completion of my work which resulted, thirty years after its inception. The birth of the Creative Act was waiting for the fast."

FOOD LIFE EXAMPLE

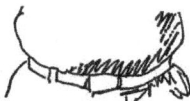

As a child she loved food and would constantly ask her mother for more to eat. "Not another thing before dinner" she was told but constantly she would beg. "I had severe food problems from the beginning." She ate herself into adolescent obesity and started dieting at 13. "At age 16 I started experimenting. I would eat a dozen donuts and a twelve-egg cheese omelet with a pound of bacon on the side. Then I would fast all day. I was amazed to see how I lost weight daily despite all that I ate. This was an amazing discovery. Although the type of food was all wrong the incredible fasting process was evident. I had found the whole key for me—it set the stage for Ramadan Fasting thirty years later. Then at 19 she "hit Atkins and all went well with cheese, meat, eggs and salads." Then she met a man who made her feel like a "murderess" for eating animals. "I became a vegetarian and it was at this point that my severe food problems began." Having given up animal protein and fat she lost her entire personality which depended on a bloodstream fed by animal foods.

When she went away to graduate school she became an anorexic. "I missed my parents—I was too immature to leave home as the family disease of alcoholism had stunted my emotional growth. I came home one weekends to rejoin the ranks of the cranks (although I loved them and miss them). But simultaneously (as often happens when girls leave home) anorexia became full-blown. Oh the cravings! They are infinite as infinite as the varieties of food. Had I just stuck to animal fat and protein I could have prevented two decades of the misery of anorexia and alcoholism. One led to another. You just can't tamper with one's protein and fat requirements without triggering real personality and identity problems." She became feeble, fretful and frail. Having lost identity her career goals began to slide.

PHONY FRUITARIANISM

This was a perfect set-up for the full-blown acceptance of fruitarianism as the only way for life, but later after two decades of low-protein and fat the body collapsed like a house of cards. "At times all I thought about was (what I needed desperately): salt and meat. Now I love salty chicken breasts: Because glucagons is elevated (without starch) I stay thin and streamlined—but I didn't know this then: I was "orthorexic": I had accepted the fruit diet whole without any reservations and no one could dissuade me from it. I had strong resolutions to maintain the fruitarian way only to binge-relapse when the meat cravings took over. With more maturity the binges stopped to be replaced by rigid routines and eating plans very anorexogenic in nature. People would say "you're so emaciated" to which I would see as a "misjudgment of purity."

All through her journals one reads "the answer to all problems is fruitarianism and more purity." She was hospitalized at times but still refused to recognize that all she needed was protein and fat--the very thing she craved. Longterm fruitarianism made her so sensitive she couldn't be around anyone and avoided groups of all kinds—family, church, neighborhood or especially triangular relationships. "Fat-famished I became frustrated, always feeling people were siding against me. I was in my own little world--inspired but with minimal outward relations." It was not until she read beyondveg.com that she recognized this as common among longterm fruitarians. "These sad stories of failure to thrive and emaciated declension was my story--everything down to the crumbling of my teeth. Even while my mouth was being restored I had staunchly defended fruitarianism to the dentist doing the work."

"Fruitarianism to an insecure person becomes a fantasy which overtakes the mind. It captures and holds one bound to an ideal--of magic castles, heaven, success, favor with man, greatness and championship. No one on earth could dissuade me for it congers up visions of another world, an ascended reality. Fruitarianism kept me 'sane' I thought, in an 'insane world.'" Alcoholism and anorexia had so warped her self-esteem that she held on to fruitarianism for dear life to the hope of future glory and relief. "It was my only lifeline and escape from hopelessness and despair. Nothing else made 'sense" despite cravings for animal protein and fat."

A COLLAPSED SHACK WITH LOW WALLS

Fruitarianism worked at first. As the body purified she became more athletic, healthy-looking and joyous. She became an outdoors person, a biker, a hiker, a yogi. She was--and still is--an early riser (2 a.m.) who worked creatively all through the day and night. She required little sleep and was far more energetic than before. "I don't think destiny could have chosen a better way to outgrow my early problems or transcend the early system. Short-term fruitarianism saved my life, served me well, but then failed—setting me up nicely to accept the exhilaration of MEAT." As a failing fruitarian she lived on a diet of non-sweet fruit (avocados, tomato, red bell, cucumber) eating a tomavo or red salad in the morning and then fasting until night—thus increasing her shaky isolation, paranoia, mood swings and denied cravings for fauna.

She was weak with no boundaries. She was unable to handle the invasions of men in the small desert town with only two cops on alert during the day. "They would come over to visit without calling first. I am a worker and this annoyed me greatly yet I had such flimsy boundaries I couldn't keep them away or at bay. I was a single weak female living alone. They knew I had a Ph.D. and felt compelled to jealously mock, invade, degrade and snatch all they could from me. It was hell on earth, a new edition but the same old template and system. I learned later that God builds a protective hedge around His own but it's broken down through sin or bad associations--the godless group. As we get older these templates must be dissolved or we die. This was the period of really finding out what people were like. I was terrified of the unwanted 'guests' in my own home but could do nothing about it until the body revived through correct diet—fauna in addition to fruit, and daily fasting. Only saturated fat—

against which we've all been hypnotized wrongly. The greatest thing was animal fat's (with lots of delicious salt's) capacity for appetite-suppression allowing me to fast for the day or for long periods. This seemed so efficient and comforting. It was the first time in my life I wasn't always hungry. Small bites of this HQ (higher quality) foods indeed brought encephalization (enlargement of the brain) as the whole height-width ratio changed and I became a longhead. Every day it's the same thing—embosomed in monotony, I excel: fasting in the evening and the next morning, fauna then the fast."

ALL DISEASE HEALED AND GOD REVEALED
Acid Reflux Cured At Last: Raw Milk

And so the late nineties were marked by inward seclusion combined with daily fasting and ascension to a much higher reality. She became "delightfully addicted" to fasting as the days were "ethereal, eternal, exquisite." She was alone in the desert, found her "peculiar niche" and was ecstatically happy there. "Each successive day on the fasting regimen new miracles occurred: Sudden, transforming, magical coincidences. Breakthroughs. Every day a new set of miracles each one higher than the previous ones."

She was now a "Christian Mystic" fasting in the desert until the "shallow façade of religiosity dropped to reveal eternity. One experiences the ALL through moral purity (whether a meat-eater or not) and self-denial which begins with fasting. This ascension to a much higher reality is a radical introduction to a brand new world. Here we see our Destiny, our potential, the beauty of the world. When not fasting--in a state of digestion--our consciousness falls to the gut and our perception of the world becomes bland, boring, mundane, stereotyped. The difference between fasting and eating is the same as winning vs. losing victory vs. defeat. To be fasting is to be sitting right in the lap of God." She ends with these words:

What a privilege to use the fail-free devices of prayer and fasting. These are devices to get to God and His infinite power. Just think: no matter what, we always have this answer to any and all problems on earth and it always works. No matter our age or circumstance we can always have the victory. The non-fasting world will simply never know the implications of this statement--nor will they ever believe its truth. Fasting is not starving--it is coming into your own with all the power of God running the show. The eater is immersed in ego which he feeds constantly. P.S. Acid reflux is cured with raw milk, meat and fasting not fruit.

Bibliography

Aiello and Wheeler in Current Anthropology 1995.

Atkins Robert. Dr. Atkins New Diet Revolution Avon Books 1992

Benoit F.et.al. Changes in body composition during Weight reduction in obesity" Arch. Of internal Medicine 63:4 (1965) p 604-612

Billings Tom. Beyondveg.com

Cassidy Claire Ph.D. in Protein Power p 401

Cockburn Mummies Diseases and Ancient Cultures in Eades p. 400

Eades Michael and Mary Dan M.D. Protein Power 1996 Bantam Books

Howard Vernon. No 50 Ways to Escape Cruel People 1981

James William. Varieties of Religious Experience 1858.

Koester, Arthur. The Act of Creation, 1962

Lovewisdom John. "Vitarianism" unpub. Manuscript 1975.

O'Dea Dr. Kerin in Protein Power by Eades and Eades p. 46

Schachter Zalman and Ronald Miller. From Age-ing to Sage-ing Warner Books 1995.

100 KAREN KELLOCK BOOKS

AFFINITY OR MISERY
AGELESS CORNUCOPIA
AMERICA AWAKE!
AMERICA'S DAFT ERA
ARTS OF PALEO FASTING
AUTOPHAGY ON CHEATERS
BACKSTABBING NEUROTICS
BETRAYAL TRAUMA
BOOMERS AND BROKENNESS
BOOT ON NECK
CHAMPION GUIDES
COMMIE NUTHOUSE
COMMIES
COMMUNIST SPIRIT
CONTAGION OF MADNESS
CONTAGIOUS MADNESS
CULTURE CLASH BASHED
DAFT LEFT
DAILY FASTARIAN
DAM RATS
DIVERSITY IS CRUELTY
E-RACE WHITE
EVIL FREAKS (Beyond Gross)
THE END OR A BEND?
FEMALE BULLIES AND FEMI-NAZIS
FEMALE CARNALITY
FEMALE DUMB DOWN
FEMALE POWER DRIVE
FEMINISM AND RUIN 1 & 2
FIX FOR MISFITS
FOOLS & TRAMPS
FREEDOM SPEAKING
FRENEMY ENABLER
FRENEMY LIAR
FRENEMY THIEF
FRENEMY TRAITOR
TRENEMY TYRANT
GENIUS IS HELD DOWN
GLOBALISLAM
GOD USES THE FLAWED
HAZE OF THE LATTER DAYS

THE HERD IN WORDS
HIX POLITIX
HOW THEY RUINED US
JUST SKIP DINNER
LE FEMME AND THE COMMUNIST SPIRIT
LIBERAL CHAOS & ROT
LIBERAL DOUBLETHINK
LIBERAL GALL 1 & 2
LIBERAL SHOVE-DOWNS
LOCK YOUR GATE
LOSERS and Femme Fatales
MANUAL FOR SUPERIOR MEN
MODERN ART FROM HELL
MOSTLY FAKE
NOTES TO CHAMPS 1 & 2
OVERCOME FRENEMIES
PC MAKES US CRAZY
PEOPLE ARE CRUEL
PEOPLE PROBLEMS 1 & 2
PERSECUTED GENIUIS
POLI-PSYCH MYSTERIES
PRETENTIOUS SLOBS
QUEEN BEE
RED NEW DEAL
RETURNING TO FIRST NATURE
SEASON OF TREASON
SEPARATE MEANS HOLY
SOCIAL HYPNOTISM
SOLITUDE SOLUTION
SUPERCILIOUS
THE SCHOOLS SCREWED EM UP
TOAD TO PRINCE
TRIALS CYCLES
TRUMP VS. GROUP
TRUST IN TRASH
THE TRUTH ABOUT PEOPLE
UNDERHEANDEDLY CLEVER
WALK TALL WITHIN WALLS
WE'RE NOT ALL ONE
WINNERS SKIP DINNER
WORK OR SMERK

AUTHOR BIO
Karen Kellock Ph.D.

Ph.D Political Psychology, UCI 1976
Post-Doctoral: UCI Medical School
Department of Psychiatry
Grants NIMH, NIAAA

Ph.D. dissertation "A Systems-Theoretic View of Pathologic Interaction" made an early mark as the "Wife of the Alcoholic Syndrome". Postdoctoral research at UCI Medical, Dept. of Psychiatry on the systems surrounding pathology on NIMH and NIAAA federal grants: The Contagion of Madness: The Psychology of Neurotic Interaction and Pathological Systems. Therapy tool Therapeutic Playwriting introduced the play Mary and Murv: Gruesome Twosomes in the Alcoholic Marriage. She taught Abnormal Psychology and Pathological Systems Theory at UC and CSU campuses and developed "the Debris Theory of Disease" in 100 books and website: (www.karenkellock.org).

www.ingramcontent.com/pod-product-compliance
Lightning Source LLC
Chambersburg PA
CBHW072129270326
41931CB00010B/1714